THE
EQUILIBRIUM
PLAN

THE EQUILIBRIUM PLAN

Balancing Diet and Exercise
for Lifetime Fitness

SALLY EDWARDS

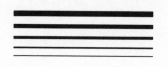

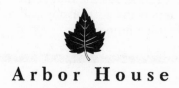

Arbor House

NEW YORK

Designed by Robert Bull

Manufactured in the United States of America

10 9 8 7 6 5 4 3 2 1

Library of Congress Cataloging in Publication Data

Edwards, Sally, 1947-
   The equilibrium plan.

   1. Reducing diets.   2. Reducing exercises.   I. Title.
[DNLM: 1. Diet—popular works.   2. Exertion—popular
works.   3. Physical Fitness—popular works.
QT 255 E265m]
RM222.2.E277   1987   613.2′5   86-32241

ISBN: 0-87795-880-7

▬▬▬▬▬▬▬▬▬▬▬▬▬

I offer the advice in this book to people who are not ill and who
have no serious medical problems that require a doctor's care. Any
readers who experience any sort of physical or mental problem
should consult a doctor immediately.

▬▬▬▬▬▬▬▬▬▬▬▬▬

To the people who have fed me and kept me racing along the roads to lifetime fitness—especially my mother, Gaye Roberts Edwards, who showed me how to stay in balance

CONTENTS

FOREWORD

by

Dr. H. ROBERT SUPERKO, MD, FACSM
Medical Director,
Lipid Research Clinic and Laboratory,
Stanford University

Americans are waging an all-out war on fat and cholesterol and Sally Edwards's *The Equilibrium Plan* gives us a powerful weapon for winning that war. Excess body fat has only recently become an obsession of the American public, but in fact it has concerned health-conscious people for centuries. Numerous books have been written extolling the virtues of this or that method of manipulating diet and calories in order to relieve the overburdened individual of unwanted body fat. Yet these books frequently neglect the equally important second half of the energy balance equation: physical activity. The role of physical activity in weight control is not a 20th-century medical revelation. In 1892 the famous physician Dr. William Osler wrote, "In some ... cases of obesity, however, this [overeating] plays no part, and the unfortunate victim may be a notoriously small eater. A second element is lack of proper exercise."

The role of proper exercise and proper diet in achieving a healthy life-style has sparked debate at many medical conferences where experts discuss the detailed physiological aspects of the subject, but Sally Edwards has put the best of what we now know together as she balances scientific accuracy, clarity of writing, and plain entertainment to explain this complex subject to anyone who wants to achieve a lifetime of fitness. Further, she places a well-aimed motivational kick to the proper anatomical region in an effort to stimulate the behavioral changes necessary to achieve a balanced diet and exercise plan for optimal health.

What goes in, must go out, or be stored, often as fat. So most dieters restrict what they eat. However, several recent scientific investigations have demonstrated that individuals can actually eat more and weigh less with the proper use of exercise! Since the quantities of food we eat have a profound effect at the cellular level and since exercise also affects the functioning of cells, proper exercise can result in permanent loss of body fat, health-ier metabolism, and long-term physical well-being. Exercise may in fact eliminate the need for dietary supplements and help prevent the dietary deficiencies caused by some diet-only weight-loss programs.

The Equilibrium Plan is particularly timely since we have embarked on a national campaign intended to lower the blood cholesterol of most Americans in order to prevent heart disease. This program, the National Cholesterol Education Program, sponsored by the U.S. government's National Heart, Lung, and Blood Institute, stresses proper diet, exercise, and weight control as the best way to prevent heart ailments. I cannot overemphasize the importance of this subject. Cardiovascular disease remains the number one killer of Americans, and it occurs in large part because of our gluttonous and sedentary life-styles. This new book, written by an exercise physiologist turned successful international ultra-athlete and businesswoman, presents a sensible and effective guide to leading a balanced and enjoyable life-style.

Sally and I have been friends and have enjoyed running together for many years. Her commitment to health and fitness originates from a place deep within her soul. She leads by example. I encourage you to not only read this, her latest book, but also to undertake the steps necessary to achieve your own personal exercise and diet plan for optimal health.

ACKNOWLEDGMENTS

My friend, agent, and collaborator, Michael Snell, guided every phase of this book's development, from helping shape my original ideas into book form to editing and rewriting the entire manuscript. Thanks, Michael, for all your hard work but especially for your sense of humor in the midst of all the pressure to meet impossible deadlines without cutting corners.

Writing a book reminds me of an aerobics workout. The writer stands in the front of the class selecting the music and orchestrating the motions, while everyone else contributes energy, enthusiasm, and sweat. The Arbor House team worked together as a synchronized team, with publisher Eden Collinsworth and editor James Raimes always pushing the rest of us to peak performances. My nutrition consultant, Elaine Moquette, BSC, MPH, RD, brought her expertise to bear throughout, especially with the nutritionally sound menu plans she designed. And Fleet Feet, Inc., contributed its art director, Ardis Bow, to provide artwork and serve as a photographer's model with fellow Fleet Feet Racer Dwight Miller. Even my key training partner, photographer Karen Coe, helped with the book—she shot all of the photos.

Friends stuck by me through thick and thin, reading and critiquing everything I wrote. Special thanks go to Theresa McCourt and typist Tracy Kelly. Thank you, too, Cheri Wolpert, John Lehrer, Greg Peterson, and Nancy Moliter.

Finally I owe a lot to my Nikes, my ten-speed, and my Speedo swimsuit, because they constantly remind me to balance my own fitness equation. I love working out, but equally well, I love good food!

INTRODUCTION

LIFETIME FITNESS

Grapefruit diets, liquid-protein diets, diets urging us to eat more fat or more carbohydrates, and quick-weight-loss diets from famous and not-so-famous doctors; fiber diets, food combination diets, and diets for allergies; blood-serum-level diets, miracle pills, and starch blockers; diets that starve us, diets that let us eat all we want, diets with easy formulas for success, and diets that claim to spot-reduce our cellulite. No wonder we're confused about how to shed and keep off unwanted pounds! But any sensible person really knows that there are two factors that determine body weight: what we eat and what we do to burn off what we eat.

I have designed the Equilibrium Plan to teach you how to balance the diet and exercise sides of what I call the fitness equation. In essence, the fitness equation states that if you are currently maintaining a stable weight you will neither gain nor lose a single ounce if you continue to eat the same way and exercise exactly as you have in the past. To lose an ounce, either you can reduce what you eat while exercising the same, or you can eat the same while exercising more. If you wish to achieve a different

1

ideal weight you can follow the Equilibrium Plan, which will have you exercising more (and more wisely), and maybe even eating more (but more wisely).

Calories measure the energy on both sides of the fitness equation. Whether you consider yourself fat or fit, whether you enjoy an outdoor job, where you get plenty of exercise, or work in an office all day only lifting a telephone receiver to your ear, you consume and expend calories. Housewives, business executives, lumberjacks, truck drivers, writers, clerks, secretaries, even world-class professional athletes, all struggle with the same equation: The calories you put in your mouth stay in your body, in the form of excess weight, unless you burn them off with activity. Regardless of your present physical condition and regardless of your life-style, work-style, eating habits, and exercise routines, the Equilibrium Plan will help you balance those calories and put you on the road toward lifetime fitness.

Balance—it works in sports, it works in business, it works in life, and it works in the war on weight. You may know a skinny person who can gobble up thousands of chocolate calories without putting on an ounce while an overweight friend watches hopelessly with a carrot stick in hand but without shedding a single ounce. If so, you've seen the fitness equation at work, but now you will understand why. The skinny eater observes both sides of the equation, controlling both intake and output to maintain a perfect balance, while the noneating overweight individual restricts eating without paying equal attention to exercise. Now you, too, can become a skinny eater by striking your own perfect balance.

Each of us has fought—and most of us continue fighting—the battle against excess weight. Unfortunately, most of us are losing. As a professional athlete and a businesswoman, I can't stand to lose, and I have dedicated a lifetime to helping myself and others become champions. Although I have designed the Equilibrium Plan for anyone who wants to look better and feel better, I have directed most of my advice to those who want to shed the 5–25 pounds that keep so many of us dissatisfied with our bodies, our bathroom scales, and our clothing size. Have you fought the battle for so long that you have resigned yourself to waving the white flag? If so, take heart, because now you can cut through all the confusion and take control of the problem.

Two fundamental rules of balance govern weight control. Rule One states that when diet calories equal exercise calories, your body weight will remain the same because you have reached equilibrium. Rule Two holds that when exercise calories exceed diet calories, your body weight will decrease, and conversely, when diet calories exceed exercise calories, your body weight will increase. If your body weight satisfies you, you can observe Rule One, but if you want to shed weight, you must follow Rule Two until you reach your ideal weight, after which you can practice Rule One for a lifetime.

To help you put these rules to work, I have designed seven practical tools which make their appearance at various stages of the book. One is the Equilibrium Plan Slide Guide, which is portable, so that you can carry it with you and take it to the supermarket or restaurant. Another is a set of menus for fourteen days. These are in Chapter 5. The remaining five tools are documents you can copy and fill out for yourself as you go through the plan: the Self-Image Evaluation Chart in Chapter 1; the Diet Calories Log in Chapter 2; the Exercise Calories Log in Chapter 3; the Equilibrium Game Plan in Chapter 6, and finally the Challenge Reward Chart in Chapter 7.

Now here is a brief preview of the plan I will be leading you through during the course of this book.

First, I will show you how to think like a winner. If you suspect that you don't think like a winner now, doing so may be easier for you when you realize that another essential ingredient of the plan is that you think in the long term. You do not have to aim at quick weight loss. Indeed, I argue strongly against your doing so. Yes, you will see improvement in just one week, but you should aim to win not tomorrow but over the long haul. It's much easier to proceed gradually and to succeed step by step. I propose not that you fall into the typical dieting pattern of winning and losing and winning and losing, but that you win permanently.

You'll start by filling out the Self-Image Evaluation Chart, comparing your present weight and general level of fitness with the image you would like to project 5 or 10 years from now or in the year 2000. On this chart you will decide on that most important figure—the number of pounds you want to lose.

Now, when you divide that figure by two, you will know how many weeks it will take you to reach your desired weight. Why?

Here's a very useful number to remember: There are 3,500 calories in 1 pound of fat, and my plan will show you how to lose 7,000 calories per week, i.e., two recognizable pounds per week. So if you want to lose 20 pounds, give yourself 10 weeks to do so, then plan to maintain your new equilibrium until the new century and beyond.

If 7,000 calories per week sounds like a lot to lose, think of it as 1,000 calories per day, which isn't a lot, especially when those calories are half diet calories and half exercise calories—not all diet calories or all exercise calories. I will show you how to reduce your calorie intake by 500 calories per day, at the same time increasing your calorie output by 500 calories. That is the bottom line of my plan for you.

But how exactly will you be doing it? As soon as you look at the Equilibrium Plan Slide Guide you will see the calorie values of a whole range of generally available foods and of an equally large range of exercise and other activities. You can start playing with the Slide Guide immediately, of course, and it will help you immediately. (For instance, a cup of popcorn cooked in oil gives you 54 calories, which you can work off at the typewriter in half an hour if you weigh 150 pounds.) But this book will show you how to put it to its very best use in a full-fledged plan that is uniquely suited to your own tastes in food and to your own choice of exercise activities—a plan that is consistent with the most up-to-date research in nutrition and exercise physiology.

Incidentally, since no two people have exactly the same lifestyle or work habits and since eating and exercise habits vary from individual to individual, the Slide Guide can only encompass a general range of foods and activities. From them you should be able to select those most suited to your own preferences. If you don't find your favorite foods or the activities you are most interested in, consult the expanded tables in the Appendix of this book.

With the Diet Calories side of the Slide Guide you can analyze your average total intake of calories per day and record the figures on your Diet Calories Log. Then you can turn to the other side of the Slide Guide to analyze your average total output of calories per day, again recording the figures in your Exercise Calories Log. The two figures you have obtained on these logs should more or less equal each other if you are in a state of equilibrium. If they don't, my book will show you how to get them to equal each other. But even before you start to make a shift in your eating and exercise habits, you will find that these figures will reveal some fascinating things about the daily functioning of your body.

Now for the shift. On the diet side of the fitness equation, I will have some advice not only on what to eat, but when, how often, and how much. I will show you what are good foods and what are bad foods (bad foods are typically those that contain too much fat, salt, sugar, caffeine, or alcohol), which foods are loaded with calories (Did you know about nuts? Look at the Slide Guide!) and I will ask that your foods generally obey the crucial 60%–25%–15% rule. That is, they should, individually or together, contain roughly 60 percent carbohydrates, 25 percent fats (far less than most Americans take in), and 15 percent protein.

To follow that rule, I will give you a great many shopping and cooking tips, and tips on eating out in restaurants. One particularly helpful tip I cannot wait to give you is this: Read labels. If the product you are buying has a label that tells you how many calories it contains and how many grams of fat, get into the habit of performing this simple arithmetic: multiply the fat grams by nine, which gives you its fat calories, then divide that figure by the total calories, which gives you its fat percentage. If it's more than 30 percent, beware!

My menus for fourteen breakfasts, fourteen lunches, and fourteen dinners obey the 60%–25%–15% rule.

On the exercise side of the fitness equation, you will learn how many calories you expend when you do absolutely nothing (this depends on the total surface area of your body and is very easy to calculate), how many calories you expend when you drive or walk to work, how many you expend on the job, and how many when you cook a meal, dig a garden, wash dishes, or jump rope. I'll give you a great many tips on how to expend more calories in each of those activities: when you wake up in the morning, when you are moving around your office, even when you are sitting at your desk talking on the telephone.

But you should also expect to start and proceed gradually with a moderate exercise program. You'll hear about the F.I.T. formula, using your heart rate to adjust the frequency and intensity and timing of whatever exercise you have chosen.

The Equilibrium Plan will move you painlessly through five levels of fitness. At the Iron level you will burn off 50 calories per workout; at the Steel level you'll move up to 100; and at the Bronze level you'll be at 200, at Silver the level 350, and at the Gold level 500. You'll start at whichever level you feel most comfortable, so you can begin experiencing the benefits of exercise right away.

Finally, this plan would not be complete without a visual record of your progress. So you'll keep a record of your weight as it changes on your Challenge Reward Chart. Watch those 2 pounds of fat coming off week after week! Watch that line plunging down to the level of equilibrium you had set for yourself, then keep to that level and enjoy a lifetime of fitness!

Over the years I myself have bounced back and forth between 115 and 140 pounds, a fact that would have surprised the spectators who watched me win the Western States 100-Mile Race in 1980. But over the years I gradually developed a deep awareness of the principles on which my own equilibrium depended, until for the last few years I have maintained an ideal weight of 125 pounds, taking in around 3,000 diet calories and expending around 3,000 exercise calories every day. I attained that goal the way you can attain yours—with this Equilibrium Plan. Good luck!

CHAPTER 1

THE FITNESS EQUATION

PREPARING FOR THE NEW MILLENNIUM

How quickly the 21st century is rushing toward us! In just a few short years we will be celebrating the turn of the century with a joyous New Year's bash. What will you bring to the party? A slightly rotund, easily fatigued, quickly aging body, or a trim, energetic, gracefully maturing you? Will you be fat or fit? Most of us would like to picture ourselves slender and fit, but unless we start making the right diet and exercise choices today, we may be sentencing ourselves to a fat new century.

I like to think of heading toward the new millennium as a sort of journey through the cosmos. To complete the trip as successfully and as healthily as possible, we must be sure that our spacesuits are lightweight and versatile. Otherwise, we will arrive at the great New Year's Eve party tired, sluggish, and overweight. Your body is like a spacesuit that you have spent decades developing and perfecting; but suppose I asked you to place a price tag on it. How much do you think your spacesuit is worth? How much do you think you would have to spend to replace it?

From the point of view of medical science, rebuilding your body with replacement parts and transplants would cost nearly $15 million. Of course, doctors can't quite do that yet because, with today's technology, they can only replace about half of the body's parts, and then only with extreme risk. If you added to the price of the body the cost of a computer with the same capacity as your brain, then your body's worth becomes incalculable, since the largest supercomputer made today (the Cray-2) sells for $45 million and lacks even rudimentary common sense. Nevertheless, let's arbitrarily price your spacesuit at $100 million. Do you treat your body as if it were that valuable, or do you live as if it were worth the mere $8.87 a junk dealer would pay for its chemical elements?

Before we learn how the Equilibrium Plan can guarantee fitness beyond the year 2000, let's agree on two points: your body is priceless and you want to enter the 21st century at your best.

If you accept the first premise, and if you set a long-term fitness goal for yourself, not only will you have taken the first crucial steps on your trip toward a new you, you will have jumped off the diet merry-go-round.

THE FITNESS EQUATION

Some 20 million of us would love to lose weight at this very moment, but an alarming percentage have been swept aboard a revolving carousel with its never-ending rotation of quick-fix diet plans, from those that promise fast weight loss with very low calorie intake to "diets" that promote gadgets, gimmicks, fads, and pills. One recent diet even proposes that certain earrings can reduce your appetite by activating acupressure points. None of these diet plans work in the long run, because when you take off weight fast, you gain it back just as fast, unless you exercise.

How many popular diets have you tried over the last 5 years? The following nine types of diets are drawn from recent lists of best-selling books.

1. High-protein diets. These diets propose that a process called specific dynamic action (SDA) will enable your digestive process to burn off extra calories. They suggest that you eat meat, poultry, seafood, eggs, and dairy products. The concept of SDA has no scientific basis, and these diets can lead to a pathological condition called ketosis from a reliance on protein and energy sources while neglecting carbohydrates as fuel. Worse, the diets are boring, hard to follow, lack essential vitamins, minerals, and fiber, and can increase blood cholesterol levels. They pose dangers for pregnant women and do not lead to permanent weight loss.

2. High-fat diets. These diets claim that the body will burn fat if it has no carbohydrates to burn, and they suggest that you eat unlimited amounts of fat and fatty foods—mayonnaise, cream, sauces. These diet plans don't allow carbohydrates. These diets are nutritionally unbalanced, high in cholesterol, and produce mostly temporary water-weight loss from glycogen depletion. Also, since fatigue results from insufficient carbohydrate intake, these diets are potentially dangerous over long periods of time.

3. Low-carbohydrate diets. Like high-protein diets, these diets insist that SDA burns more calories than are contained in the food you eat. They recommend a consumption of unlimited amounts of protein, again with no carbohydrates. The same objection applies to these diets as to high-fat diets. Since insufficient amounts of carbohydrates produce fatigue, low-carbohydrate diets are potentially dangerous over long periods of time.

4. Gimmick diets. One such diet suggests that eating food in certain combinations and at certain times of day will result in weight control. Another proposes that the body is allergic to certain foods and reacts by gaining weight. Another recommends that you eat fruits and vegetables and undergo massage and heat-lamp treatment, guaranteeing removal of your fat deposits (cellulite). Another requires that blood serum levels be measured regularly. The truth is that no combination of foods or eating-time sequences produces weight loss, so-called cellulite cannot be removed by a combination of diet and massage treatments, and taking regular blood samples has no scientific validity as a weight-loss technique.

5. Single-food diets. One of these suggests that you eat unlimited amounts of grapefruits with specific foods, such as eggs, and another, that you drink unlimited amounts of juice. The problem, of course, is that you cannot obtain necessary nutrients if you only eat a single food item. Such diets are boring, nutritionally deficient, and fail to change poor eating habits.

6. Pill diets. Dexedrine, Dietac, Dexatrim, VitaSlim, and Appedrine are examples of diet pills containing appetite suppressants. These propose that you can kill your appetite with amphetamines or other "natural" substances, such as an extract from raw beans. Amphetamines, however, are addictive; they cause appetite suppression and exhilaration. As diuretics, they produce fluid loss, but they also cause insomnia, hypertension, depression, tremors, and nervousness.

7. Formula diets. One of these advises you take in only 300 liquid calories a day; another advocates 900 to 1,000 calories in a canned drink. Because they reduce the basic number of calories to a figure below that required to sustain your basal metabolic rate (see page 63), such diets can be dangerous, often resulting in nausea, hair loss, constipation, and cramps.

8. Very-low-calorie diets. Extremely low-calorie diets are simply near-starvation plans. Typically, they set 500- to 1,000-calorie days; some even alternate several weeks of severely low-calorie intake (600 calories per day) with a week of low-calorie intake (1,200 calories per day). Such a regimen can create extreme imbalances in your metabolic system. It can also lead to bingeing, headaches, lack of energy, and other problems.

9. Fasting or starvation diets. One of these allows no calories from solid food, recommending only liquids and some noncalorie foods. Another suggests that you wire your jaws shut, so you can only take in liquids. Such programs can be extremely dangerous and may lead to anemia and loss of lean body muscle needed for functioning. They lack vitamins, minerals, and fiber.

Clearly all of these diets pose problems, but another recently popular one does not. A vegetarian diet suggests that you eat only foods from plants, or plants plus dairy products, or plants, dairy products, and eggs. These are the best of the popularly promoted diets. A properly balanced vegetarian diet can be an excellent and healthy way to lose weight. It is safe and provides nutrients. Studies have shown that in the United States vegetarians outlive meat eaters, who are prone to heart attacks, by an average of ten years.

If you have followed more than one of the nine problematic diets, you have been riding the merry-go-round, whether you know it or not. To stop the merry-go-round you must abandon the illusion of quick weight loss and adopt, instead, a longer-range view, one that begins with your long-term self-image and a steady concern not only for what you eat (diet) but also for what you do (exercise) to prevent the calories you eat from turning to fat. In short, you must balance the fitness equation, which states that whatever excess calories you eat turn to fat unless you burn them off. While some diet books may pay lip service to the importance of burning off calories, they nearly all focus on rapid weight loss. But to achieve such loss, you must shed fat, water, and *muscle tissue* while dieting. Given the fact that muscle loss reduces the body's ability to move about, we can see why proponents of rapid weight loss play down the importance of exercise.

Not surprisingly, popular exercise books do the reverse, focusing on workout programs without paying equal attention to the proper fuels the body needs to get the most out of exercise. Getting into and staying in shape, however, depends as much on what, why, when, and how much you eat as it does on the specific forms of exercise you adopt.

My Equilibrium Plan will show you how to lose *any* amount of weight gradually (2 pounds per week) and to keep it off permanently by balancing your own fitness equation with a sensible diet of good foods and a regular, moderate regimen of exercise. Everyone—from the presently fit to those who wish to shed unwanted fat—can find his or her own equilibrium point, that point at which healthful diet and exercise combine for a lifetime of fitness. This book will help you reach that point.

EVERYBODY CAN BE A WINNER

Are you a winner, with a spacesuit worth millions, or a loser, with one worth pennies? Like most people, you probably classify yourself somewhere in between. While you may jog 20 miles a week or attend aerobic dance classes twice a week, you may also wish you could shed or rearrange a few pounds. Or you may have won the battle of the bulge last spring as you dieted and exercised your way into summer fun, only to lose it again when the temptations of Thanksgiving turkey and Christmas pudding rolled around. Then again, you may compete—as I do—in ultra-athletic events, such as triathlons and 100-mile races, but despite your regular workouts and a carefully controlled diet, you still worry about achieving the correct balance between what you do and what you eat. The Equilibrium Plan can solve any of these problems. In the battle *against* weight and *for* fitness, everyone can win.

Regardless of your current image of yourself as a winner, a loser, or in between, your future image depends on what I call self-worth building. Even athletes struggle with it. Take the example of my friend John Bair. In 1979, John, 146 pounds of lean mass, ran beside me in the Western States 100-Mile Race. Then, over the next several years, he gradually stopped exercising, until he seldom worked out more than once a week; but since he maintained his accustomed diet, John gained fat and lost muscle until his spacesuit slowly ballooned. When his weight hit 190 pounds, he had exited the winner's circle completely.

John thought he was a triple loser. He was losing the weight war, he was losing a great deal of self-esteem, and he was losing the admiration of his athletic friends. But John was also lucky, because deep inside his oversized spacesuit and in the minds and hearts of his friends, he still retained the potential to become a winner again. When he decided to place a higher premium on his self-worth and set his sights on a fitter future, he had embarked on his road to a new equilibrium.

Today, John thrives at his ideal weight of 155 pounds, cherishes a rebuilt self-image, and enjoys the admiration of all his friends. You, too, can become a winner if, like John, you dedicate yourself to self-worth building. *You are what you eat and what you do, but you are, first of all, what you think.*

Like all long-range endeavors, Self-Worth Building works best if you break it down into a few clear, logical steps.

- Define your current self-image.
- Establish your ideal self-image.

- Project your new self-image 15 years into the future.
- Design a short-term nutrition plan that will quickly reinforce your ideal self-image.
- Simultaneously engage in a short-term exercise plan matched to your diet plan.
- Gradually develop a long-term equilibrium plan that will put you where you want to be in the year 2000.

We'll look at the last three steps later in this book, but for now let's talk a little more about the first three. How do you picture yourself at the moment? A full-length mirror or a bathroom scale or a tape measure will tell you part of the story, but you might also consider inviting your friends, family, and loved ones to tell you honestly what they see. Since the admiration of friends—the third component of triple winning—both motivates and rewards us, it can really help to involve others in our self-image evaluations. Next, imagine your ideal self, the one you hope to be maintaining 15 years from now. If you become aware of the differences between your present and projected self-image (in terms of appearance, weight, measurements, and the views of others), you can obtain here a very clear quantitative and qualitative idea of what you wish to accomplish in the long run. If you do not know your percent body fat and percent fat-free weight, for instance, Chapter 3 will show you how to calculate these quite easily.

The Self-Image Evaluation forms that follow will help you complete the first three steps listed above. I have filled one out for a hypothetical person, and I have left one blank for you to use yourself. You may find it difficult to project a clear self-image 15 years into the future. Just take the time and let your mind open to imagine what you would love to be like. Then fill in the form.

I keep my own evaluation on my refrigerator door, where I see it every morning. Next to it I have taped a photograph of a red Ferrari, because in 15 years I still want to look like a lean and fast race car, powered by high-octane fuel and capable of sweeping the field at Le Mans. Kids who like to hang posters of their heroes, from champion athletes to rock stars, on their bedroom walls, not only hero-worship these people, they also visualize becoming like them when they grow up. You can remind yourself of who you are and who you want to be when you "grow down." Regardless of your own personal ideal, place representa-

Self-Image Evaluation

<u>Today</u>	<u>The Year 2000</u>

Your age today: **43**   Your age in the year 2000: **56**

Weight: **177** pounds   Weight: **150** pounds

Measurements in inches: **15½** neck, **47** shoulders, **43** chest, **36** waist, **40** hips, **26** thighs, **14** upper arms

Measurements in inches: **15** neck, **48** shoulders, **40** chest, **30** waist, **36** hips, **22** thighs, **16** upper arms

Percent body fat: **25%**   Percent body fat: **15%**

Percent fat-free weight: **75%**   Percent fat-free weight: **85%**

Appearance: Appearance:

How others see me: _____   How others see me: _____

pudgy, low-energy   **slender, good muscle tone**

How I see myself: _____   How I see myself: _____

fat, slow, lethargic   **confident, strong**

Regular exercise routine: _____   Regular exercise routine: _____

running   **running, bicycling, weight lifting**

Personality: Self-defined: _____   Personality: Self-defined: _____

quiet, dependable   **confident**

Defined by others: _____   Defined by others: _____

introverted, low-energy   **gregarious, enthusiastic**

tions of it wherever they will do the most good: on your refrigerator door, over your bathroom scale, beside your dressing-table mirror, near your exercise clothes and equipment, in your wallet.

If you place current photos of yourself and your Self-Image Evaluation next to your goal pictures, you can look in the mirror 30 days, 6 months, a year, or a few years from now to see how much progress you've made.

Self-Image Evaluation

Today | The Year 2000

Your age today: _____

Weight: _____ pounds

Measurements in inches: _____ neck, _____ shoulders, _____ chest, _____ waist, _____ hips, _____ thighs, _____ upper arms

Percent body fat: _____%

Percent fat-free weight: _____%

Appearance:

How others see me: _____

_____

_____

How I see myself: _____

_____

_____

Regular exercise routine: _____

_____

_____

Personality: Self-defined: _____

_____

_____

Defined by others: _____

_____

_____

Your age in the year 2000: _____

Weight: _____ pounds

Measurements in inches: _____ neck, _____ shoulders, _____ chest, _____ waist, _____ hips, _____ thighs, _____ upper arms

Percent body fat: _____%

Percent fat-free weight: _____%

Appearance:

How others see me: _____

_____

_____

How I see myself: _____

_____

_____

Regular exercise routine: _____

_____

_____

Personality: Self-defined: _____

_____

_____

Defined by others: _____

_____

_____

FIVE KEYS TO LIFETIME FITNESS

You will also profit from learning about how formerly fat people have lost weight. In the past, researchers studied thin and fat people to learn how they got and stayed that way, but they seldom studied those who made dramatic changes one way or the other. Only recently have researchers begun to focus on people who have won the permanent-weight-loss war, shedding and keeping off 10 to 30 pounds of weight for more than 5 years. After studying the attitudes, eating behaviors, exercise activities, caloric and nutrient consumption, life-styles, and thought processes of successful dieters, I have detected a few "secrets" and "tricks." I have concluded that in the final analysis five common threads run through the stories of successful long-term weight loss.

People who have moved from heavy to thin, from fat-full to fat-balanced have invariably developed the following:

1. A clear self-image with high self-esteem. Nothing contributes more to fitness success than a clear self-image and high self-esteem, but developing that sort of confidence and pride takes a lot of effort. Most overweight people think fat, while they would have a better chance to lose weight by thinking thin, and most nonexercisers have trapped themselves with a nonathletic self-image. But all of us can be thin and athletic, provided we define ourselves that way. *Think thin.* Your Self-Image Evaluation and your personal representations of your ideal self can start you on the right track toward increased confidence and pride. No one else can do it for you, although your friends, relatives, and fellow dieters and exercisers will help motivate and reward you.

2. Sound eating habits. Successful weight loss depends on developing three basic food habits. First, eat when you are hungry, not when your appetite calls. Hunger signals the body's need for nutrients, while appetite signals your emotional need for taste satisfaction. Second, know what you are eating, and follow the rules of healthy nutrition. Learn to tell the difference between good food and bad food, always weighing the costs and benefits of what you eat. Third, don't be obsessed by food. Learn the principles of good nutrition, and pay attention to what you eat. Don't compulsively count calories; take pleasure in eating. This doesn't mean that you can go on an eating binge, but it does mean that thin people enjoy eating as much as fat people. However, they do not eat beyond their needs. Instead, they achieve an ongoing balance between what they eat and what they do to burn off calories.

3. Regular exercise routines. The formerly fat have discovered the secret of exercising off excess weight. You must exercise moderately every day, making your workouts as much a part of your day as your mealtimes. Exercise should become a permanent part of your daily life-style, and missing a workout should bother you as much as missing a meal. Successful dieters pay equal attention to both sides of the fitness equation.

4. Self-motivation. Long-term success hinges on continuing motivation, and motivation depends on a system of rewards. Give yourself a pat on the back when you lose a few pounds of fat, or, better yet, give yourself a tangible gift, such as theater tickets or a pair of walking shoes. Eventually, you'll receive the most valuable reward of all—a feeling of personal power that comes from fitting into stylish clothes, weighing exactly what you want to weigh, looking and feeling your best, and enjoying the respect and admiration of others. Most important, you'll reduce your risk of disease and degeneration, and you'll live longer.

5. High-energy life-styles. Long-term winners of the weight war free themselves from stress and such self-indulgent abuses as chemical and substance dependence. You must learn how to control more than just your body weight. You'll find that a high-energy life-style will help you develop healthy relationships with relatives, friends, neighbors, and fellow fitness-conscious individuals.

These five keys, working together, will put you in the ranks of triple winners. Winning the game of life is like winning any other game. In competitive sports, winners always prepare themselves thoroughly, play by the rules, and visualize a successful outcome. In the diet game you must do the same. But, like the successful athlete, you must also become a risk taker.

This is a very important point. Most of us have become accustomed to taking risks in our lives, be they in our personal relationships or in our business or career endeavors. In my own case, every time I compete in a marathon or a triathlon I risk my reputation as an athlete, and sometimes I even risk injury by pushing my body to its limits. Every time I open a new Fleet Feet athletic sports store I risk a great deal of time and money, and also my business reputation.

But then think about the far greater risks we take with our lives when we *don't* do something sensible, such as controlling the balance between eating and exercise. Every extra pound you carry in body fat reduces your quality of life *now* and may shave months off your life span, and every day you fail to exercise or to eat properly may increase your chances of getting heart disease, hypertension, or cancer. Those are the kinds of risks we should all avoid. So, what do you risk when you decide to balance the fitness equation? Well, you run the risk of failure. But if you've been riding the diet merry-go-round, you've already failed, probably more than once, and you might even suffer a setback or two after you begin the Equilibrium Plan. However, failure, like thinness, is more a state of mind than a physical condition. If you succeed for a while, then fall off the wagon and gain back a few pounds, don't despair. Risk again.

CHAPTER 2

THE DIET SIDE OF THE EQUATION

CREEPING OBESITY

Jack Taylor and I have been close ever since we first started dating in college. I was 19 years old when I met Jack, and he was my first true love. Do you ever look back at old photographs and wonder that you ever looked like that? I do, especially when I see that freshman-year college snapshot in which I wore penny loafers complete with the penny, plaid pleated skirt, a white blouse, and my kite-shaped sorority pin. I was skinny as a rake, and so was Jack.

During the next four years we both changed as we immersed ourselves in campus life at the University of California at Berkeley. I was active in student politics, marched to protest the war, and boycotted my graduation ceremonies to protest the National Guard's gunning down and killing James Rictor, a fellow student, during the demonstrations. Jack played rugby and intramural football, stood fast with his fellow ROTC cadets, and signed up as a forward observer in Vietnam after his graduation. I, too, volunteered to go to war, as a Red Cross worker.

Although we went our separate ways after the war, Jack and I stayed in touch and developed a strong long-distance friendship. While I was beginning my professional sports career and launching my chain of Fleet Feet stores, Jack completed two years of postgraduate school, then started working at a publishing house. He continued to play recreational rugby until he permanently damaged his shoulder, then his exercising routines quickly gave way to a demanding desk job.

A few years ago Jack sent me a picture of himself at the beach. What a change. As so often happens to men around the age of 32–35, he had started to put on weight. His muscles had atrophied from inactivity and had become filled with fat. He looked pretty good on the outside, but having known him in peak condition, I could tell he was experiencing white-collar sedentary deterioration. At age 34, Jack was halfway up the corporate ladder and halfway down the overweight staircase. He was suffering from creeping obesity, steadily gaining about 2 pounds a year, and whenever he went on a diet, he somehow ended up heavier than before. He had become living proof that diets don't work. Then, for his 35th birthday, I gave him a present that he says changed his life—a gift certificate to be fat-tested underwater. After the test he was shocked to discover that although his total body weight had increased only 10 percent over his weight in college, his percentage of fat weight had gone up 20 percent. That's when he went on the Equilibrium Plan.

The laws of thermodynamics determine how energy gets translated from one form to another. When the human body absorbs food energy into the bloodstream, that energy goes to one of two places: to little energy factories in our cells called mitochondria or to storage. *A body in equilibrium balances energy intake with energy output, but a body that takes in more than it expends accumulates fat in cells throughout the body.* In Chapter 3 you will learn how to build more energy factories in order to burn more calories and create higher levels of energy, and you will see how the body fills up its fat cells, but at this point simply bear in mind that an imbalance leads to fatness. And being fat hurts. On the outside, it hurts your looks. On the inside, it hurts your health, clogging your arteries, restricting your breathing, and contributing to a variety of diseases.

Within 6 months, Jack fixed his problem permanently, and

today he eats good foods and good calories. He eats whenever he wants and as much as he wants of a high-carbohydrate, low-fat diet, and he combines exercise with other calorie-burning activities for an hour a day to burn off everything he eats. Not only does he have more energy for his career, his body looks good to himself and his friends. We'll take up the exercise side of the fitness equation in Chapter 3, but for now let's focus on the food side.

CALORIES FROM CARBOHYDRATES, FATS, AND PROTEINS

Before you begin any new diet, you must ask one basic question: What does the diet allow you in terms of nutrients and calories? Remember, a workable diet must be healthful, balanced, and serviceable for a lifetime.

Four times I have finished the Hawaiian Ironman Triathlon among the top five. To do so, I had to complete the 140.6-mile race (a 2.4-mile swim, a 112-mile bike ride, and a 26.2-mile marathon) as fast as I could, but without damaging my health. By the time I finish an Ironman competition, I have burned over 9,000 calories. During each of the three times that I have run (and one time won) the Western States 100-Mile Race, I have burned over 17,000 calories.

If I were following one of the 300-calorie-a-day diets, that 9,000-calorie Ironman would have burnt up a full month's worth of eating. Obviously, had I adhered to any sort of very-low-calorie diet, I would have lacked the fuel to complete even the swim part of the race. On the other hand, if I ate the calories needed to compete in endurance contests when I manage my business, travel from coast to coast, or sit glued to my word processor, my spacesuit would start to resemble a blimp.

So do I count calories? Sure I do, but it comes automatically now as I adjust my eating habits to match my level of activity. You will not want to or need to count calories forever, but you nevertheless should learn to recognize and evaluate them.

A calorie (technically termed a kilocalorie) is the unit that measures the energy value of both food and physical activity. It is the amount of heat needed to raise the temperature of one gram of water by one degree Celsius. For example, if a poppy-seed bagel contains 161 calories, the energy trapped inside the bagel would change the temperature of 161 grams of water one degree Celsius, and a 110-pound person who ate that bagel would have to take a brisk half-hour walk to burn off those calories.

You may be interested in how scientists measure the calories in different foods. They use a device called a bomb calorimeter. If we place that poppy-seed bagel inside the bomb calorimeter's enclosed chamber with charged oxygen gas and ignite the bagel-oxygen mixture with a spark, the mixture explodes. An inner liner insulates the chamber. This water-filled insulating bag absorbs the heat from the burning bagel, while a thermometer measures the rise in water temperature. We call the released heat the heat of combustion, which is exactly what the body experiences when it ingests, digests, and then exercises off those 161 calories.

An average 5' 5" woman requires and burns about 2,100 calories per day. An average man (who is 4 inches taller with 10 percent more muscle weight than a woman) burns about 2,700 calories per day.

Calories come from only three nutrient sources—carbohydrates, fat, and proteins—and are used for fueling the muscles,

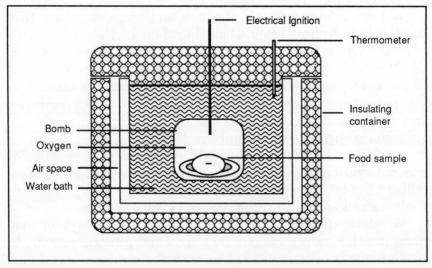

The Bomb Calorimeter

storing energy needs, and building body tissues. (Alcohol also contains calories but is not considered a nutrient source.) We use grams or ounces (there are 28.4 grams in one ounce) to weigh each of these three nutrients, then we convert them into calories.

Your body burns each of the nutrients in different ways. On the average, a gram of carbohydrate delivers 4 calories, a gram of fat 9, and a gram of protein 4. These whole numbers, called the Atwater general factors, have been used by nutritionists for nearly 50 years to represent the energy available to the body from the three sources of calories.

Despite continuing debate among nutritionists over the correct percentages of carbohydrates, fats, and protein a healthy diet should contain, a general consensus has formed called the 60%–25%–15% rule. The safest, most healthy, most properly balanced diet should consist of 60 percent calories from carbohydrates, 25 percent calories from fats, and 15 percent from protein.

The National Research Council has set recommended daily allowances (RDA) of carbohydrates, fats, and proteins, but I suggest that you set for yourself daily amounts that reflect the 60%–25%–15% rule (except for pregnant women, who should eat 30 grams (1.06 ounces) more protein per day, and lactating women, who should eat 20 grams (.7 ounce) more protein per day).

If you are going to eat a 1,500-calorie diet, then the 60%–25%–15% rule would apply as follows:

Carbohydrates .60 × 1,500 calories = 900 calories divided by 4 calories = 225 grams or 7.95 oz carbohydrate

Fats .25 × 1,500 calories = 375 calories divided by 9 calories = 42 grams or 1.48 oz fat

Protein .15 × 1,500 calories = 225 calories divided by 4 calories = 56 grams or 1.98 oz protein

Would a 1-cup scoop of vanilla ice cream fit the 60%–25%–15% rule? At the risk of getting a little mathematical for a moment, let's look at how a nutritionist would answer that question.

A 183-gram, 6.6-ounce scoop of typical (not "extra rich") ice cream contains 37 grams of carbohydrate, 19 grams of fat, 8 grams of protein, and 120.6 grams of water (which isn't figured into the calculations, because water contains no calories).

If a gram of carbohydrate equals 4 calories, we then multiply 37 times 4 to calculate that our scoop of ice cream contains 148 calories worth of carbohydrates. Similarly, the fat, with 9 calories per gram, contributes 171 calories, while protein, with 4 calories per gram, adds only 32 calories.

Our scoop of vanilla ice cream contains a total of 349 calories. Of these, 42 percent comes from carbohydrate (148 divided by 349), 49 percent from fat (171 divided by 349), and 9 percent from protein (32 divided by 349). Bad news for ice cream lovers: clearly, vanilla ice cream is a 42%–49%–9% bad food and flunks the 60%–25%–15% test!

What if you add an ounce of hot fudge, a dollop of whipped cream, and a handful of crushed walnuts to the ice cream? Wouldn't you have to be a mathematician to figure out the food values and calorie count? Yes. If you scrupulously counted your calories yourself, you would spend so much time calculating that the ice cream would melt and you wouldn't have time left to eat it, much less exercise it off.

But don't despair. The Equilibrium Plan Slide Guide and the Appendix will help you quickly and accurately determine the calories of most of the foods common to the American diet. It can become a permanent, and eventually intuitive, tool for determining both food calories and the exercise needed to burn off those calories. Meanwhile, though, you should know how to separate the good foods/good calories from the bad foods/bad calories.

BAD FOOD/BAD CALORIES

In the Equilibrium Plan, the bad foods will not surprise you: They include fats, sugars, salt, caffeine, and alcohol. Each of these can create an imbalance in the fitness equation. Let's look at each of these foods in turn.

What one word makes us weight-conscious folks shudder more than any other? *FAT.* Obviously, if we don't want to get fat, we must control the calories that add fat to our bodies. Given the fact that a sound long-term diet should include about 60 percent carbohydrate, 25 percent fat, and 15 percent protein, my definition of a good food is that it adheres to the 60%–25%–15% rule, and of bad food that it doesn't.

Most foods don't perfectly fit the 60%–25%–15% rule, and in fact many violate it. It is the violators that are potentially bad, and can easily unbalance your dietary equilibrium. To avoid those potential dangers, consider them in a sense "bad" from now on and use them with caution.

As in basketball, the tallest player and the one hardest to defend against, FAT, dominates the action. Although we only need between 135 and 225 calories of fat daily to supply us with the three essential fatty acids (i.e., those needed to sustain healthy metabolism), the average American overdoses on fat tenfold.

As we noted above, vanilla ice cream gets nearly 50 percent of its calories from fat and therefore qualifies as a bad food. Other popular foods with more than 50 percent of fat calories are potato salads, made with ½ cup mayonnaise (58 percent), pork chops, even trimmed of fat (73 percent), whole milk (51 percent), a fast-food-franchise fried drumstick (53 percent), and a popular chain's breakfast sandwich or hamburger with cheese (51 percent).

Most of us don't deliberately choose to eat fat-full foods. In fact, when queried, most overweight people can't tell you how much fat they consume, especially in the form of meat, nuts, and dairy products. This lack of knowledge about the hidden fats hurts the unknowledgeable dieter. To boost your own awareness, consider the sampling of foods in the following table that contain over 50 percent fat.

FOODS WITH TOTAL CALORIES FROM FAT IN EXCESS OF 50 PERCENT

Food	Percent Calories from Fat	Food	Percent Calories from Fat
Butter, salted	99	Potato chips	63
Cream cheese	91	Corn chips	60
Coffee with cream	90	Fried liver	59
Avocado	85	Bass, baked and stuffed	58
French salad dressing	83	Pound cake	57
Hot dog	79	Veal roast	55
Roasted peanuts	77	Chocolate candy bar	55
Cole slaw	74	Creamed fish	53
Raw egg	67	Whole milk (3.5 percent fat)	51
Imitation whipped topping	64		

As if fat weren't bad enough all by itself, it tends to be associated with cholesterol. High consumption of saturated fats increases blood cholesterol levels and thus the risk of heart disease. Saturated fats, which are fats that are solid at room temperature, such as lard and shortening, aren't always easy to recognize. Some plant fats, for example coconut oil or palm oil, contain no cholesterol yet fall into the saturated group and raise your cholesterol levels. Advertisers may claim "100% cholesterol-free vegetable shortening," but they don't tell you that saturated vegetable fats will also cause your cholesterol levels to rise.

To make fats more appealing, merchandisers also like to label them "hydrogenated," a process that turns liquid fat into solid fat, thus improving its shelf life. It doesn't improve human life, though, because the oil has merely been changed from polyunsaturated fat to a partially saturated fat.

If you have to eat fat, then select foods that are low in cholesterol and that contain polyunsaturated or monounsaturated fats. When using cooking oils, select olive oil, safflower oil, soy oil, corn oil, or sesame oil.

Next, fat's best buddy, simple sugar, plays a mean game with his high level of energy. Refined sugars, which include all types of table and cooking sugars (white sugar, powdered sugar, high-fructose corn syrup, honey, etc.), have earned a starting position on the bad food team because, unlike the complex carbohydrates (the starches and sugars found naturally in fruit and milk products), they can be quickly absorbed into the bloodstream without being first broken down in the stomach. That isn't good.

If you dump such sugar into your bloodstream in large concentrations, you will experience a sugar rush. At first, you will feel on top of the world, but as your body rushes insulin into the blood to metabolically handle the sugar, you start to suffer the sugar blues. Sugar bouncing can wreak havoc on your physical and mental health, and, what's worse, refined or simple sugars also consist of blank, or empty, calories (i.e., they offer no nutrients and provide no minerals or vitamins). When you eat extra calories in bad food sugar, your metabolic process stores the sugar molecule as a fat or glycogen. This conversion of sugar into fat is the body's system of storing excess calories for future conversion into energy when the body makes physical demands to burn calories.

The next bad food is salt, which breaks down into sodium and inactive chloride. Every body needs sodium to keep water floating in the cells and bloodstream, but too much of it can increase the risk of high blood pressure, heart attack, kidney failure, and stroke. Thus, we should limit our use of salts, both on the table and in the foods we eat. Even if you use the salt shaker sparingly, you may inadvertently indulge in other high-sodium condiments, such as ketchup, steak sauce, MSG, Accent, soy sauce, and pickles, as well as salt-coated foods, such as peanuts, pretzels, and potato chips.

Caffeine can really fake you out. A member of the family of compounds called xanthines, caffeine functions as a stimulant, causing rapid increases in pulse rate, blood pressure, and the amount of free fatty acids circulating in the bloodstream. Again, you may already be restricting the amount of coffee you drink, but you may unwittingly be consuming large amounts of caffeine in cola drinks, tea, chocolate, cocoa, and certain over-the-counter drugs. If you want a false high, drink a can of cola, but if you want a real high, take your body for a stroll in the fresh air or walk up and down the stairs in your building. Sure, your body can handle small amounts of bad foods, but the stimulant that your body really wants is exercise, exporting rather than importing drugs.

The final player is a big one: alcohol. Not only can it harm your body (mental incapacitation, depression, cirrhosis), it can hurt others as well (vehicular deaths, homicides, suicides). A depressant and a diuretic (it dehydrates you), alcohol also overworks your liver, which tries to remove it from your bloodstream. Like sugar, alcohol feeds you blank calories. A daily excessive consumption of alcohol, whether with the lower concentrations in beer or the higher ones in hard liquor, can disrupt every aspect of your future self-image.

GOOD FOODS/GOOD CALORIES

To beat the bad foods you can field the good-foods team, which includes five key players:

- High carbohydrates/low fats
- Fiber

- Fluids
- Vitamins
- Minerals

And good foods play by two rules:

- Variety
- Balance (in calories and nutrients)

If we wish to fuel ourselves with all of life's natural nutrients, we should build variety into our diets and exercise regimens. Variety not only sustains our motivation to stick with a lifetime health commitment, but it also allows us to modify our programs to reflect aging processes and changing life-styles.

Good foods also recognize the importance of balance. Not only should we eat a balanced diet in terms of the 60%–25%–15% rule, we should daily eat one food from each of the six modern food groups: meat or fish, dairy products, cereals/grains, fruits, vegetables, and the convenience foods (those manufactured by processors or restaurants). Each food group contains foods with varying percentages of carbohydrates, fats, and proteins, but you should emphasize those that obey the 60%–25%–15% rule. A balanced diet also includes at least the minimum RDA of vitamins and minerals, as well as plenty of water, which contains no calories. Finally, a healthful diet depends on eating the right things in the right proportions for the right reasons at the right times.

High Carbohydrates/Low Fats

Carbohydrate-rich foods, such as spaghetti, noodles, beans, potatoes, fruits, vegetables, and rice, generally cost less at the supermarket than fat-rich foods, such as steak, sausage, eggs, bacon, and butter. To obtain energy, you can put twice the volume of complex carbohydrates at 4 calories per gram into your system as you can of fats at 9 calories per gram. For these reasons alone, a high-carbohydrate, low-fat diet makes the most sense—and it reduces your grocery bill.

But what about protein? Of course, you do need protein in

your diet, but the amount necessary for an active life-style has been overrated, overadvertised, and touted to death. Exercise does not increase your protein need—it increases your carbohydrate need. However, we have been seduced by marketers to believe that we can develop beautifully toned bodies by drinking protein-rich whole milk (51 percent calories from fat), protein-rich blenderized eggs (67 percent fat-full calories), or taking amino-acid supplements or even protein powder dissolved in whole milk. Well, fine, but what do we do with all the extra protein we obtain from such a diet? In some cases our bodies convert it to glucose and *fat*.

One last word about protein. Animal protein sources are usually high in fats and calories. Take a moment to list what you consider to be high-protein foods. A 6-ounce (untrimmed) steak contains 805 calories, with 83 percent of those calories in the form of fat. Eggs? A two-egg omelette with 1½ ounces of cheese contains about 361 calories, 71 percent from fat.

Fiber

Fiber is a nondigestible carbohydrate with few, if any, calories. Until recently, most people ignored fiber as an inconsequential part of their diets, but current studies indicate that it actually helps to reduce constipation, prevent hemorrhoids, reduce blood cholesterol levels, and lower the incidence of death from some types of cancer and heart disease. It provides bulk with almost no calories.

The average American consumes only about 10–15 grams of fiber per day but should be taking in three times that amount, or 30–45 grams. Our low fiber levels generally indicate that we eat too much fat. High-fat dairy products and meats lack fiber. Fresh fruits and vegetables, dried fruits, and nuts and seeds contain a lot of fiber, and you can obtain even more from unprocessed whole-grain foods, such as brown rice, oats, cornmeal, and wheat flour. Bran is loaded with fiber and can make very appetizing cereals, breads, and muffins.

Because different foods contain different types of fiber, we can't rely on just one fiber-rich food. We need all types for good health, but basically we want to build two main sources into our diets:

1. **Fiber that doesn't dissolve in water.** These fibers include wheat, grains, vegetables, and fruits. They increase bulk in the intestines and remove food waste from the intestines more quickly. They also reduce constipation and protect against appendicitis, gastrointestinal disease, and colon cancer.
2. **Fiber that forms a gel in water.** These fibers include citrus fruit, legumes (beans), oats, barley, some vegetables (e.g., corn). They slow the emptying of food from the stomach into the intestines, as well as the absorption and entry of carbohydrates into the bloodstream. They also help reduce serum cholesterol.

The following foods offer the highest fiber content.

HIGH-FIBER FOODS

Food	Fiber (grams)
Cereals	
All Bran, 1 cup	22.50
Wheatena, 1 cup cooked	3.30
Vegetables	
Artichoke hearts, cooked, 6 ounces	24.00
Beans, great northern, 1 cup cooked	15.00
Beans, kidney, 1 cup cooked	19.40
Broccoli, 1 cup cooked	9.40
Celery, diced, 1 cup raw	7.00
Peas, green, 1 cup cooked	17.00
Spinach, 1 cup cooked	11.30
Tomatoes, 1 cup cooked	5.74
Yams, 1 cup cooked	7.80
Fruits	
Apple, 1 medium	4.28
Blackberries, fresh, 1 cup	10.50

Blueberries, fresh, 1 cup	4.93
Fruit cocktail, in juice, 1 cup	4.28
Prunes, dried, 5	6.75
Raisins, 1 cup	11.20
Raspberries, fresh, 1 cup	9.10

Whole Grains, Breads, Pasta, and Other Grains

Bran, corn, 1 ounce	18.53
Brown rice, 1 cup cooked	4.50
Buckwheat flour, 1 cup	8.00
Bulgur wheat, 1 cup cooked	7.10
Cornbread, 1 serving, from mix	4.00
Dark rye flour, 1 cup	12.00
Oats, rolled, dry, 1 cup	5.70
Pasta, whole-wheat, 1 cup	4.94
Soy flour, low-fat, 1 cup	12.00
Whole-wheat flour, 1 cup	11.50

Although such foods as lettuce, mushrooms, and onions have only small amounts of fiber, you can make a traditional salad a higher-fiber food by adding kidney beans, and vegetables like broccoli and artichoke hearts.

Fluids

"Water, water everywhere, but . . ." Possibly the most versatile but overlooked player on the good-food team is that ubiquitous fluid we take so much for granted. The body's natural lubricant, water facilitates movement and acts as a solvent for the body's normal chemical reactions. If we reduced a human being to his or her basic elements, we would wind up with a few ounces of inexpensive chemical elements and several gallons of water. Yet, few of us drink the 8–20 or so 8-ounce glasses of water we need every day. If we did, we would not only quench our thirst and lubricate our bodies, we would be putting into our stomachs a calorie-free substance that can suppress our appetites for richer fare.

Vitamins

We obtain the number four good-food group, vitamins, in the form of organic substances derived from living materials. These organic substances can cause a lot of controversy. Some people, such as the chemist Linus Pauling, promote anti-cold and other health benefits of vitamin C. Nutritionists agree that there are 13 vitamins and that they come in two forms—fat-soluble (A, D, E, K) and water-soluble (the eight B vitamins and C). To meet the U.S. RDA standards, all the required vitamins together only add up to about an eighth of a teaspoon per day. That's how little we really need. But vitamins are essential for the processing and metabolism of foods, and they help our bodies manufacture blood, hormones, genetic material, and nervous-system chemicals.

You don't need to take a vitamin supplement if you can eat a balanced diet and if you aren't exposed to toxins, stress, drugs, cigarette smoke, alcohol, processed foods, or air pollution, if you don't use birth control pills and certain prescription and over-the-counter drugs, if you are not elderly or don't display certain disorders, such as chronic infections or cancer, if you aren't healing from surgery or injury, or if you don't have to follow some specific diet for health reasons. But if you are a city dweller who eats on the run, must ride on airplanes, or works in an office with cigarette smokers, you might consider hedging your bets with a daily multivitamin. Keep in mind that while you cannot easily overdose on water-soluble vitamins, such as C, you can take too many fat-soluble ones, such as A.

Minerals

The only inorganic player on the team is minerals. As with vitamins, all bodies require small amounts of minerals. Minerals also come in two types: trace minerals and macrominerals. The body needs extremely tiny amounts of trace minerals but larger amounts of macrominerals. While the trace minerals—chromium, copper, fluorine, iodine, iron, manganese, molybdenum, selenium, and zinc—make up only .01 percent of your body weight, the macrominerals—calcium, chloride, magnesium, phosphorus, potassium, sulfur, and sodium—make up 4 percent.

Minerals enhance many vital, even critical, functions throughout the body, but megadoses of minerals can actually poison the body, so you should take extreme care not to take more than the necessary amounts, which you will obtain naturally from a balanced diet. Iron and zinc can be exceptions, and your doctor can tell you whether or not you need supplements of these in your diet. The sodium in salt is a member of the mineral family, and if you eat excess quantities, it becomes a bad food.

Two minerals demand special attention—calcium and iron. Calcium represents 2 percent of your body weight, and your body stores 98 percent of its calcium in the bones, with the remaining 2 percent split evenly between the teeth and the soft tissues in your body. It's the one macromineral that can require supplementation, especially for mature women. If your body lacks a sufficient supply, hormones will remove calcium from your bones and use it for other life-sustaining roles, and, as a result, you will suffer from bone deterioration. This condition, osteoporosis, commonly afflicts women endurance athletes, the elderly, and postmenopausal women. Bone-loss experts recommend a daily minimum of 1–1.5 grams per day of calcium. To meet this requirement, you may need more than supplements because to absorb 1 gram of calcium a day, you would have to take six pills that when stacked are a half inch tall, each the diameter of a quarter. Fortunately, many foods, such as dairy products and sardines, are rich sources of calcium.

Iron deficiency doesn't really affect your blood so much as your general energy level; and Popeye was wrong, too. Spinach provides less iron than many vegetables like lima beans, beets, parsley, tomato puree. Iron deficiency anemia, which may take years to develop, does lead to fatigue, weakness, pallor, and shortness of breath. Infants, vegetarians, adolescents, endurance athletes, and menstruating women frequently lack the proper levels of dietary iron. In fact, as many as 5 percent of American women suffer iron deficiency. Again, overdoses of iron can damage the liver, pancreas, and heart.

This completes the good-food lineup. These foods play fair and follow the rules of the game: balance and variety. They demand your total daily respect and should form the basis for your healthful diet.

How do you substitute good foods for bad foods? Experience makes a big difference. My dad was a World War II pilot and war hero who made the Navy his career. My three older brothers and I grew up on TV dinners, macaroni and cheese, and canned beef stew. Like most kids, we shunned vegetables, especially Brussels sprouts and spinach. As a result, I annually ate my weight in sugar, enjoying its rush, and I worshiped red meat as king and whole milk as queen of the dinner table. When we asked, "Hey, Mom, what's for dinner?" she always answered with the name of the meat she had prepared.

But I learned to debunk the myths of the all-American diet when I trained for athletic competition. The more I trained, the more my body naturally craved good foods. By working out we get in closer communication with our own natural needs and gain confidence in rejecting the ever present media messages. As I started to compete in ultradistance running events, I realized I was running farther and farther away from mom's "home cooking," a combination of processed foods, red meats, and fat-full dairy products.

By the time I was regularly entering 100-mile races, I had completely traded high fat for high complex carbohydrates because my muscles demanded them for the tough trails I traveled. Today, when I head out for a "century" bike ride, I carry only three bananas (complex carbohydrate/low fat), three water bottles (fluids), and a $5 bill to purchase some fruit juice and rice cakes (variety and balance for when I stop). I devour foods filled with fiber and bulk as I spin over the miles and the hills in the gold country above Sacramento.

EQUILIBRIUM PLANNING AND SHOPPING

You now have all the general information you need to construct for yourself the sort of healthful menus you will find in Chapter 5. For example, if you are a typical woman needing 2,100 calories per day, your menus should consist of 60 percent carbohydrates (315 grams or 11.13 ounces or 1,260 calories, of fruit, vegetables, and grains), 25 percent fat (58 grams or 2.05 ounces or 525 calories, of meat, eggs, dairy products, seeds, and nuts), and 15 percent proteins (79 grams or 2.79 ounces or 315 calories, of lean meat, fish, eggs, and milk products). Likewise, if you are a typical man on a 2,700-calorie daily plan, your menus should balance with 1,620 calories (405 grams or 14.26 ounces) of carbohydrates, 675 calories (75 grams or 2.64 ounces) of fat, and 405 calories (100 grams or 3.52 ounces) of protein. You should always include in your diet a variety of foods from each of the six modern food groups:

1. Meat and fish: high in protein, iron, zinc, and fat calories (*Caution:* may also contain high levels of saturated fat and cholesterol).
2. Dairy: high in protein, calcium, and riboflavin and fat calories (*Caution:* may be high in saturated fat and cholesterol).
3. Grains: high in carbohydrates, iron, niacin, fiber, and vitamin B_1 and other minerals and vitamins.
4. Fruits: high in carbohydrates and vitamins A and C.
5. Vegetables: high in carbohydrates and essential vitamins.
6. Convenience foods: 20th-century foods that are manufactured by processors or restaurants. (*Caution:* may contain high levels of fat calories, salt and sugar.)

Fruits and vegetables are important not only because they provide a great deal of volume compared to fatty foods, but also because they contain many fewer calories. For example, a typical weight-stable woman who eats 2,100 calories a day entirely from the fruit and vegetable food groups, choosing only carrots, apples, bananas, and potatoes, would need to eat (and imagine yourself eating these volumes) the following amounts each day: 50 dark orange carrots, 6 apples, 2 bananas, 5 potatoes (portion size: 1 6-inch carrot = 20 calories; 1 apple [3 per pound] = 70 calories; 1 medium banana = 100 calories; and 1 medium potato [3 per pound] = 90 calories).

A calorie measures potential food energy, regardless of whether it comes from carbohydrates, fats, or proteins. The 349 calories from a 1-cup scoop of vanilla ice cream equals the calories from 17 carrots. When you consider them in this light, you can see why ice cream is a bad food and carrots are a good food. Incidentally, I choose dark orange carrots because they provide lots of vitamin A (the darker the orange pigment, or carotene, in the carrot, the more vitamin A it contains), and carotene itself may help us reduce the risk of cancer.

A 6-inch carrot has 1 gram of protein, 4 grams of carbohydrates, and no fat. To calculate the calories contributed by protein, fat, and carbohydrates, we multiply the 4 grams of carbohydrate by four calories and 1 gram of protein by four calories. Voilà, a 20-calorie carrot!

To determine the calorie percentages contributed by carbohydrates and proteins, divide their quantities by the total number of calories. The carrot gets 16 out of its total of 20 calories from its 4 grams of carbohydrates. Thus, the carrot contributes 80 percent of its calories in the form of complex carbohydrates and 20 percent in the form of protein. Does the carrot meet the 60%–25%–15% rule? Magnificently. It weighs in at 80%–0%–20%.

Does the carrot include any bad calories? No, carrots do not contain refined sugars, alcohol, caffeine, salt, or high fats; they do contain high carbohydrates, low fats, minerals, fiber, and water. They are nutrient-dense. Eat them with apples and a slice of unbuttered bread, and you have added variety and balance to your winning team.

Every ten years 6,000 new food products come onto the market, offering a bewildering array of choices. Imagine the potential confusion! But you can cut through all the confusion when you shop by playing the label game. By federal law, each packaged or processed food must carry an ingredient label, which lists each ingredient, starting with the ones most dominant by weight and ending with the lightest. If you see sugar listed first, that means the food contains more sugar by weight than any other ingredient.

Let's look at a typical ingredient label for a popular name-brand cookie:

Made from: unbleached wheat flour, sugar, partially hydrogenated vegetable shortening (soybean and/or cottonseed and coconut oils, palm kernel oil), sweet chocolate, nonfat milk, whole eggs, cornstarch, egg whites, salt, vanilla extract, baking soda, lecithin, and peppermint oil

---

From this information, we can conclude that the product contains mostly unbleached wheat flour (a fancy way of saying white flour), followed by sugar and fats. It's a bad food.

Here's an example of an ingredient label from a so-called natural breakfast cereal:

> **Ingredients:** Wheat bran with other parts of wheat kernel, sprouted wheat, sprouted barley, raisins, and yeast

The product contains lots of wheat bran, other parts of the wheat kernel, and sprouted wheat but no sugar, no fat, and no salt. It's a good food.

As a rule, the longer the ingredient label, the poorer the quality of the food. As you walk down the grocery aisles, read every label before you place it in your grocery cart. Before long you will be selecting more good foods than bad.

Food additives cause a lot of confusion because of their long and questionable-sounding names. Some of the additives are good for us, and some are dangerous. Manufacturers add them to food to change its flavor, shelf life, texture, appearance, and nutritive value. (They add green color to mint ice cream to give it a minty look.) Scientists have not yet figured out all the pluses and minuses of additives, but testing on many of those generally recognized as safe (GRAS) has resulted in many questionable additives remaining on the approved list: BHT (a preservative), caffeine, MSG (a salt), waxes, saccharin, synthetic food colors (Blue No. 1, 2, Citrus Red No. 2, and half a dozen others), and nitrites and nitrates (which color, preserve, and flavor meats). Fortunately, any potentially dangerous additives are generally found in foods that are bad for other reasons (high in fat or sugar or salt), so you can avoid them fairly easily. Snack foods, artificial beverages, packaged cakes, processed meats, sausages, and candy often contain lots of additives and few nutrients.

Though not required by law, many food manufacturers stick a nutrient information label on their products. These labels recommend a suggested serving size, tell you the weight of protein, carbohydrate, and fat in grams, and calculate the calorie content per serving size. Most will list the percentage of U.S. RDA per serving for many vitamins and minerals. If the RDA is 100 percent, then the product contains all of the nutrients needed daily by people over the age of four.

Can you trust a name-brand canned soup that claims to be "natural" as a good food source? Let's apply the rules to see if this "creamy natural asparagus soup" qualifies:

Ingredients: Chicken stock, asparagus, cream, butter, wheat flour, water, salt, cornstarch, whey, sugar, and white pepper.

The label also tells us that a 1-cup, or 8-ounce, serving contains 200 calories and 14 grams of fat if combined with milk. To tally the percentage of calories from fat, you multiply 14 grams of fat per serving by 9 calories per gram for a total of 126 calories from fat. Next, divide the 126 fat calories by the total number of calories (200) to determine that the serving would give you 63 percent fat calories. This soup ends up flunking the 25 percent fat test.

What else does this label tell us? Always check the sodium levels. This one provides 855 mg of salt, four times the 200 mg of salt you lose each day in sweat and not much less than the 1,000- to 3,000-mg maximum recommended per day. This "natural" soup is a veritable salt mine.

Inside your supermarket the bad foods sit right beside the good ones. Good-food shopping usually calls for shopping the perimeters, where the "live" foods are stored—fruits, vegetables, grains, meats, and dairy products. In the middle of the store you usually find the packaged and processed "dead" foods. You should spend most of your time on the perimeters of the supermarket, but you will find other "healthy aisles" in a typical store.

In the middle, grocers often shelve reduced-calorie or fat-free foods, such as special salad dressings, whole-wheat flour, popcorn, whole-grain cereals, dried noodles, water-packed tuna, fruits canned in their own juice, frozen unsweetened juices, and whole-wheat bread. Make a mental chart of your own local market, planning your shopping course to avoid those aisles filled

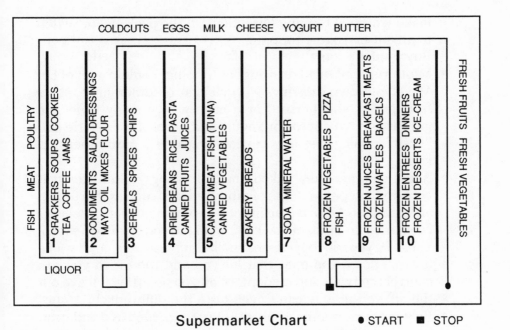

Supermarket Chart   ● START   ■ STOP

with high-fat and/or low-nutrient foods. Here are some other tips on how to become a smart shopper.

- Read the label. Multiply the grams of fat by 9, and see if the figure you get (fat calories) is less than a quarter (25%) of the total calories on the label. If it's more, beware.
- Avoid hydrogenated and saturated fats; instead, choose unsaturated vegetable oils, such as monounsaturated olive oil or polyunsaturated safflower oil.
- Switch to nonfat or low-fat milk and milk products. Gradually begin introducing milk at 2 percent fat, later replacing it with skim milk or milk at 1 percent fat. You can give skim milk more body and flavor by stirring in a little nonfat dry milk, which also provides additional calcium.
- Buy sherbet, frozen yogurt, ice milk, or frozen fruit bars (some are now 100% pureed unsweetened fruit) instead of ice cream.
- Don't buy nondairy creamers and whipped toppings, which contain palm oil and other saturated fats. Use low-fat milk or nonfat dry milk in place of creamers; use nonfat dry milk to

make whipped topping (directions on the package) or switch to a fruit or yogurt topping.

- Buy nonfat yogurt.
- Most prepared salad dressings or toppings contain a lot of fat. Make your own dressings with vinegar or lemon juice, other fruit juices, and herbs. For a cheesy or creamy style, use low-fat cottage cheese or yogurt and herbs. Low-calorie and "fat-free" salad dressings are now available in most supermarkets.
- Avoid commercially baked goods, frostings, and mixes that contain high percentages of saturated fats, such as shortening and palm oil. Animal crackers, fig bars, ginger snaps, molasses cookies, plain graham crackers, or angel food cakes are exceptions. If you do buy mixes, including pancake and waffle mixes, choose the ones that let you add the fat so you can control the types and amounts of oil you use. (If you leave out the oil, you usually can't even taste the difference)
- Rely more on nonmeat sources of protein, such as dried peas, beans, and tofu.
- If you do eat beef, choose rump roast instead of prime rib and slice it thinly.
- Instead of regular hamburger, buy ground round (the label will say "extra lean").
- If you or your family loves fat-rich luncheon meats or hot dogs, try turkey or chicken frankfurters and low-fat processed meats instead. However, gradually reduce the number of times you serve these foods.
- Cut back on red meat (beef, lamb, and pork) and use chicken, turkey, fish, or vegetarian entrées instead. There are some excellent vegetarian cookbooks.
- Don't buy prebreaded foods and commercial coating mixes, which usually contain saturated fats. You can make your own coating with plain bread crumbs, Parmesan cheese, and herbs.
- When reading labels, look for key words that indicate added fat like shortening, lard, palm or palm-kernel oil, coconut oil, egg and egg-yolk solids, whole-milk solids, imitation chocolate, milk chocolate, butter, or animal fat. An unidentified vegetable fat, oil, or shortening usually indicates either palm or coconut oil (saturated fats).

YOU ARE WHEN, WHY, AND HOW MUCH YOU EAT

A complete diet plan involves more than wise shopping and appropriate menus, because it should take into account not only *what* you eat but when, why, and how much. By studying those who have succeeded at weight control, we can gain some valuable ammunition for winning our own wars on weight. Successful weight loss requires a certain style of eating.

When?

Eat when you're hungry. Hunger is not the same as appetite. Appetite represents a psychological desire for food, while hunger signals the body's need for nutrients. Pay attention to your body's communication. Hunger signals come from the stomach, while appetite signals come from the brain. If you think you've lost touch with your hunger mechanism, wait until your stomach growls before you eat, and if it rumbles frequently, eat smaller meals more often to keep your blood sugar at the right level.

Why?

Emotions such as frustration, depression, anxiety, and boredom govern most overeating. That's another reason why learning to use exercise or other tension reducers to handle stress should become an integral part of your diet. Turning to food when you're emotionally upset can ruin your chances of achieving equilibrium. Eating doesn't address the real problem—it may even aggravate it by making you feel another emotion: guilt. Guilt undermines the confidence you need to gain control over your eating habits.

Eating bad foods can create guilt, too, although you can actually eat some bad foods without throwing yourself out of equilibrium. Usually, when I eat a bad food, I do so consciously. For example, the day following my second-place finish at the 1986 Ironman-Canada Triathlon, the North American championships,

I craved peach pie à la mode. The host city, Penticton, is the peach capital of Canada, and throughout the 112-mile bike leg and the 26.2-mile marathon we passed miles of peach trees. I scored both the peach pie and the ice cream at a family restaurant, and it tasted so great I ordered seconds. Each helping fed me well over 1,000 relatively blank calories, but I left the restaurant with a smile and sense of satisfaction.

A blank, or empty, calorie is still a calorie of energy and still counts in the weight balance, but you can indulge, say, with ice cream or a chocolate milk shake as long as you do so only occasionally. However, the smart dieter substitutes the good for the bad. First, decide what you are craving. At the Ironman-Canada I craved something creamy and laced with sweet fruit. I could have eaten fresh peaches and ice milk instead of the double helping of peach pie à la mode I wolfed down. Let's say you crave something bready or starchy, such as a croissant. Think of a substitution—a plain bagel or a bran muffin that was not prepared with a lot of butter. Chocolate attracts most of us, but satisfy your craving with a little cocoa powder on a good food, or add cocoa to nonfat or low-fat milk. If you dream about bacon or some other greasy food, eat the leanest you can find. If you thirst for something sweet, have some fresh or frozen fruit, fruit juice, or blend any of those with some sparkling water and ice to make a frozen delight.

Eating patterns vary with each person. Can you describe yours? Do you skip meals, then pork out late at night? Do you eat unconsciously in front of the TV? Have you ever eaten when you were bored or upset? Are you a snacker? Do you continue to eat even after you feel full?

Analyze your own pattern, noting what triggers your appetite and how you might satisfy it better. The following tips will help:

- **Eat slowly.** Put your fork down between every bite. Time yourself at the table. Slow yourself down by eating with your unaccustomed hand. Try chopsticks. Talk between every bite.
- **Eat by feel, not by the clock.** Your hunger mechanism does not obey a time clock. Just because the hands of the clock indicate noon, that doesn't mean you must automatically eat lunch. The best time to eat is when you feel hungry.

- **Eat regularly.** On the other hand, skipping meals or following erratic meal schedules causes a biochemical chain of disasters to occur in your metabolic system. Chronically overweight people regularly skip meals to "save" calories. Doing so, however, only makes them eat more calories later.
- **Drink fluids.** A glass of water 10–20 minutes before mealtime will help you feel fuller. Drink water between mouthfuls during meals to slow the eating process.
- **Snack early in the day.** If you are in the mood for something crunchy during the day, munch on carrot sticks or popcorn.
- **Plan ahead.** Construct menus and shopping lists. Chop raw vegetables ahead of time and pop them into plastic bags for quick salads. Cook double batches of good foods and freeze them for a later meal.
- **Stop and think before you eat.** By taking some time to assess your appetite and hunger, you can begin to tell the difference between the two. If you pause to reflect, you might not eat at all.

Appetite can be triggered by cues hidden deep in our past experiences. Did your mother insist that you finish everything on your plate, whether you were hungry or not? We associate people, places, and events with specific foods: Sporting events go with peanuts and beer; a trip to the coastline demands fish and chips; having the flu earns hot soup and love.

Appetite can also be stimulated by external cues, such as TV commercials, billboards, or magazine ads. The clock triggers appetite. So do certain smells. Can you stroll past the popcorn concession at the movie theater without your mouth watering? Unless you learn to recognize these environmental cues, you will have a hard time modifying your eating behavior.

You want to take control of your eating behavior. Ask yourself questions about why you eat. Do you respond to the sight and smell of food? Does the thought of eating cause you to eat, or do you allow something in your environment to stimulate your appetite? Do you inadvertently eat while doing something else, such as reading the paper?

Other people can drive us to eat; a spouse's cravings can become our own as we stop to share a doughnut or a hot-fudge sundae. In any case, food never solves problems, and it won't ever improve your relationships with your boss, spouse, or in-laws.

How much?

If you eat lots of food, it doesn't necessarily mean you eat lots of calories. If you could eat one head of iceberg lettuce, you would ingest less than 100 calories and it would provide a considerable amount of volume. You would feel full, and it would take a long time to eat all that greenery. A portion size of one food item may contain very different amounts of calories than a portion size of another.

We want to focus on how many calories we eat. The Equilibrium Plan Slide Guide will provide a quick and easy way to know the number of calories in hundreds of foods. With it you can reduce your caloric intake across the board by cutting back on individual portion sizes. But for now, consider these suggestions for reducing the amount of food you eat:

- Freeze single portions of main courses so you can reheat them later for a quick, portion-controlled meal.
- Fill a small plate rather than a large plate. Even if you go back for seconds, the portions will be smaller.
- Use calorie-controlled frozen entrées. Frozen entrées are included among the menus in Chapter 5.
- Buy smaller portions. Instead of making a whole pie or batch of cookies, buy one cookie or one slice of pie. If you do bake, freeze portions for later consumption.

THE ART OF HEALTHFUL COOKING

Now here are some tips for the weight-conscious cook. You'll see that the principles you should apply to your shopping apply to the way you cook the food once you have brought it home.

- Instead of cream cheese, try low-fat cottage cheese blended with a little low-fat plain yogurt. Add chopped chives, dried vegetables, or herbs for a spread for bagels or sandwiches.

- Use nonfat yogurt in place of mayonnaise for tuna or chicken salad mixtures.
- When using yogurt in cooking, add a teaspoon of cornstarch per cup to prevent curdling.
- Cut back on egg yolks. If the recipe calls for four eggs, try using four egg whites (a great source of protein) but only two yolks.
- You can use egg substitutes in many recipes.
- When cooking or baking, experiment by gradually reducing the amount of fat in a recipe. You can usually reduce the amount by a third to a half without changing the taste or texture of the food.
- When making puddings, cream pies, or cream sauces, use skim milk.
- Open-faced pies have less fat than two-crust pies. A deep-dish apple or pear crisp made with a topping of dry cereal offers far less fat than a two-crust fruit pie.
- Trim visible fat from meat before cooking.
- Remove skin and fat under the skin from chicken, turkey, and game birds.
- Leave vegetable skins on. They usually contain many nutrients and fiber.
- Use liquid oil instead of solid shortening.
- For 1 ounce of baker's chocolate, substitute 3 tablespoons of cocoa powder plus 1 tablespoon of low-fat margarine.
- Use low-fat yogurt for half of the oil in an oil and vinegar salad dressing recipe.
- Put nonfat or low-fat yogurt and low-fat cottage cheese into vegetable dips instead of sour cream (add dry soup mix to nonfat yogurt for a great vegetable dip).
- Choose white meat over dark, but select dark vegetables over light. A chicken breast has slightly fewer calories than a chicken leg. Dark carrots offer more nutrients than pale orange ones.
- Use meringues as toppings on fresh fruit for dessert.
- When preparing a meat sauce or stew, brown the meat separately and drain the fat before reheating.
- Thicken sauces by reducing them. Instead of adding butter and flour, use potatoes that are lower in calories as thickeners.
- Bake, broil, or roast instead of pan-frying meats. Use a rack

when roasting so fat can drain off. To avoid dryness, baste with lemon juice, broth, wine, water, or tomato sauce.

- Serve smaller portions of meat (stews loaded with vegetables, chili made with beans, pasta dishes, and so on).
- To grease your pans, use cooking sprays instead of bottled or canned shortening or oil.
- Use nonstick skillets and baking pans
- Sauté foods in wine, juice, tomato sauce, or soup broth.
- Try not to combine two naturally fat foods (e.g., adding cheese to a roast beef sandwich, butter to a croissant).
- Add less fat at the table. Season with herbs or spices instead of butter, margarine, cream sauces, or gravies. Be aware of these table fats and how much they cost you. For example, 88 percent of the calories in cream cheese (99 calories per ounce) come from fat. On the other hand, Neufchâtel cheese offers 81 percent calories from fat and 74 calories per ounce.

THE EQUILIBRIUM PLAN SLIDE GUIDE℠

It's time for me to introduce the Slide Guide that accompanies this book. Although you can use it seriously and casually on its own, I have designed it as an integral part of the Equilibrium Plan.

Most fitness experts say that if you focus on calorie counting when you diet or exercise, you may inadvertently ignore other equally important aspects of fitness, such as variety, vitamins, minerals, and moderation. I hope it is clear how important I view those other aspects. I would also hate to think that you would put off the enjoyment of food or the fun of exercising by having to spend too much time punching keys on a calculator.

However, quantifying your intake and output of calories will, I believe, prove quite enlightening. By doing so, you'll learn about the nature of diet, exercise, and yourself. And the Slide Guide will make it easy.

Here's how to use it. Since the fitness equation has two sides, so does the Slide Guide. On the diet side, you will find all six modern food groups and many common food items. The groups are Meat and Fish, Dairy Foods, Fruits and Nuts, Breads and

Cereals, Vegetables, and Convenience and Other Foods, each of which includes over twenty representative food items.

To make the Slide Guide plan more useful, I have added a code to each food, identifying it generally as a good food or a bad food. Good foods offer high nourishment and low fat percentages, and I've awarded them a clear circle. Bad foods represent nonnutritious calories or high fat percentages, and they receive a cross. Between the two extremes lies a whole range of foods that may not be great but aren't terribly bad either. A black square identifies these not-so-bad foods:

CODE: ○ Good foods
         Nutritious, and 30 percent or less calories from fat
CODE: ■ Not-so-bad foods
         Nutritious but 30–60 percent calories from fat
CODE: ✕ Bad foods
         Nonnutritious, or 60 percent or more calories from fat

Using the diet side of the Slide Guide involves five easy steps:

1. Select the food item.
2. Determine the food group.
3. Pull the arrow in that food group to the food item.
4. Read the nutrition, fat, and calorie contents in the window.
5. Determine the total number of calories by multiplying the number of calories in each portion by the number of portions.

Let's see how it would be used. Suppose that for breakfast you ate two pieces of whole wheat toast, a slice of cantaloupe, and a bowl of cooked oatmeal with skim milk but no sugar. Locate "Whole wheat bread" under the Breads and Cereals group, moving the arrow to show the calories in the window. Do the same for "Oatmeal, cooked." Next, move the arrow to the Fruits and Nuts group for "Cantaloupe," then find the value of skim milk the same way under Dairy Foods.

All the items in the breakfast menu represent good foods (i.e., they provide nutritious calories and 30 percent or less fat calories). If you could afford more fat calories, you might even add a bad food to this meal, such as a tablespoon of peanut butter on the toast. You would find that in Fruits and Nuts, moving the arrow to "Peanut butter" reading the number in the window, and dividing that number by 32 (32 tablespoons in one cup). Now you can total the breakfast's calories by taking the number of portions into account:

BREAKFAST CALORIES

Food Group	Food Item	Code	Amount	Calories	Portions	Total
Breads and Cereals	Wheat toast	○	1 slice	65	2	130
Breads and Cereals	Oatmeal	○	1 cup	145	1	145
Fruits and Nuts	Cantaloupe	○	1 cup	48	1	48
Dairy Foods	Skim milk	○	1 cup	86	1	86
Fruits and Nuts	Peanut butter	✕	1 tablespoon	46	1	46
Total:						455

If you frequently eat a food that does not appear on the Slide Guide, such as kiwi fruit, you should be able to find it in the Appendix of this book. Alas, even the enlarged list there cannot contain every conceivable food.

YOUR PERSONAL DIET CALORIES LOG

Now you can use your Slide Guide to fill out your personal Diet Calories Log. Over the next week, choose three days—one weekend day, one day early in the week, and one day toward the end of the week—and record everything you eat from the moment you awake until you fall asleep. Immediately after you eat (that's no more than 10 minutes), record everything you eat. If you wait longer than that, you won't be as accurate. If a day turns out to be atypical, choose another that more accurately reflects your daily habits. In addition to foods and calories, you will also want to keep track of the *quality* of the food you eat. Notice that the log contains spaces for food quality codes as well as quantities and calories.

On the next page you can see how Jack Taylor began his Diet Calories Log for a typical day, during which he ate breakfast at a fast-food restaurant, lunch at the corner delicatessen, dinner at home, and a few snacks in between. Note that he found some of the calorie values in the Appendix of this book.

On the following page you will find a blank Diet Calories Log,

DIET CALORIES LOG

NAME: Jack Taylor   **DATE: September 13, 1987**

	Code	Serving Size	Calories	Number of Servings	Calories
Breakfast					
Fast-food egg in muffin	×	1	327	1	327
Orange juice	○	8 oz	111	1	111
Coffee with cream	×	3 Tbs cream	60	1	60
Total breakfast calories					498
Lunch					
Small salad w/blue cheese dressing	×	1 cup lettuce, 2 Tbs dressing	160	1	160
Hot dog	×	1	183	1	183
Hot dog bun	○	1	150	1	150
Iced tea	○	12 oz	0	1	0
Potato chips	×	2 oz	326	1	326
Total lunch calories					819
Dinner					
Raw celery	○	1 stalk	5	1	5
Boiled medium potato with 1 Tbs butter	■	1	145 & 108	1	253
Fish stick	×	1	50	5	250
Chocolate brownie	×	1	86	1	86
Red wine	×	8 oz	151	1	151
Total dinner calories					745
Snacks					
Fruit pie	×	1 slice	403	1	403
Popcorn cooked in oil, with butter	×	1 cup	54	4	216
Soda pop	×	12 oz	136	2	272
Total snack calories					891

Ratio good-to-bad foods: 4:12
Total calories for day: 2,953

which you can copy or photocopy so you will have a handy supply
for recording what you eat. The purpose of keeping your own log
is to determine your average daily calorie intake. You need to
know the quantity and quality of your daily calorie intake to be
able to add or subtract from it.

DIET CALORIES LOG

NAME: _____   DATE: _____

Meal	Code ○ good foods ■ not-so-bad foods × bad foods	Serving Size	Calories	Number of Servings	Calories
Breakfast					
———	———	———	———	———	———
———	———	———	———	———	———
———	———	———	———	———	———
Total breakfast calories					———
Lunch					
———	———	———	———	———	———
———	———	———	———	———	———
———	———	———	———	———	———
———	———	———	———	———	———
Total lunch calories					———
Dinner					
———	———	———	———	———	———
———	———	———	———	———	———
———	———	———	———	———	———
———	———	———	———	———	———
Total dinner calories					———
Snacks					
———	———	———	———	———	———
———	———	———	———	———	———
———	———	———	———	———	———
Total snack calories:					———

Total calories for day: .... ——

Comments: _____

You might keep a few other points in mind as you complete your Diet Calories Log:

- Be sure to add all beverages (alcoholic and nonalcoholic), snacks, candies, and the like to your count.

- Include any spreads or sauces you put on your food, such as jam, butter, gravy, cheese sauce, ketchup, and sour cream.
- If the serving amount listed on the Slide Guide does not match the amount you ate, adjust the value of your portion size accordingly.
- Always remember that the percentage of fat calories is very important. Periodically add up the grams of fat you eat every day, multiply by nine, and divide that figure by total number of calories. Check that your percentage of fat calories does not exceed 25% of your total calories.

Now it's time to take a look at the other side of the fitness equation.

CHAPTER 3

THE EXERCISE SIDE OF THE EQUATION

THE YO-YO EFFECT

Jody Carper and I became close friends when we served together in Vietnam during the height of the war. It was 1970, and America had just invaded Cambodia. Although Jody and I did not participate directly in combat, we waged another kind of war, working for the Red Cross to implement a special recreation program designed to raise plummeting troop morale.

I was 21 years old and armed with my new master's degree in exercise physiology from the University of California, Berkeley. Jody, five feet nine and extremely attractive, was a graduate of the University of Maryland. We shared a lot besides our age, trim figures, and dedication to our new jobs. We developed a deep bond as we witnessed endless scenes of brutality.

The war ended, and over the next 10 years Jody and I saw little of each other. But after she married her soldier boyfriend, they visited me in California and decided to stay. Settling into the comfortable California life-style, Jody began to experience creeping weight gain (about 5 pounds a year). This troubled her, but she said her bad knees wouldn't let her exercise.

I taught school for 3 years before starting my own sports business, Fleet Feet. I had continued exercising and began to enter competitive footraces in 1973. By 1976, I had run my first 26.2-mile marathon, and three years later I had won an ultramarathon footrace, the Western States 100-Mile Race. During the next four consecutive years I finished in the top five in the Hawaiian Ironman Triathlon, maintaining my weight at a fit 120 pounds, with 10–12 percent body fat.

By now Jody had admitted her weight problem. Unable to get it under control, she said she followed the "see-food diet." She'd laugh about it: "Whenever I see food, I eat it." Actually, she embarked on five or six new diets each year, abandoning each one fatter than when she had begun it.

Jody went through a series of unfulfilling jobs, then enrolled in a night-time law school program. Over the next 3 years of sitting her way through work days and school nights, she accumulated another 30 pounds. Jody wanted to land a job with a top law firm after graduation, so she joined a popular weight-control group. She still avoided exercise, but the group support helped her shrink from 210 pounds to the perfect 125 pounds she had weighed as a 21-year-old Red Cross worker in Vietnam. Jody looked beautiful as she walked up to the podium to receive her law degree, and her future seemed assured when she accepted that dream job.

Five years later Jody again tipped the scales at 200 pounds. She was unhappy and embarrassed. I suggested she start working out. "But, Sally, I have bad knees," she insisted. "I *can't* exercise the way you do." Well, she could not compete in ultra-athletics immediately, but she could declare war on her weight by taking that first crucial step toward balancing her fitness equation: a sensible exercise program designed for her particular situation, bad knees and all.

I urged Jody to picture her body as a long, slender balloon. "When you blow into it (i.e., put food in your mouth), the balloon expands into a bigger, rounder shape unless you let that extra air out (i.e., burn off the excess weight with body movement)," I told her. "Once your balloon has gotten plump, you can only get it down to normal size by creating more outflow than inflow. Yes, you could stop blowing it up (i.e., restrict the diet side of the equation, as you have done in the past), but you will gain no lasting benefits unless you start letting out some air (i.e., increase the exercise side)."

Most Americans experience creeping weight gain as they age, but they don't lose sleep over this year's extra 5–10 pounds because the increase occurs over a relatively long 12-month period. We've all attended reunions with friends or relatives only to surprise them with remarks like, "My, how much you've changed!" Change just creeps up on us. But creeping changes become painfully obvious when you see people only occasionally, especially when they have gained 20–25 pounds. In Jody's case, she had gained 85 pounds (17 pounds a year, or 1.5 pounds a month) before she turned to a support group for help. When she did so, a restricted-calorie diet helped her shed her unwanted weight, but when she stopped dieting, she found her body ballooning out again. While Jody really believed that the diet worked for her because she did lose weight, in fact it failed to give her more than the short-term illusion of success. As a result, she had fallen victim to what I call the yo-yo effect, a physically unhealthy and sometimes psychologically devastating cycle of weight loss/weight gain.

According to a number of studies, *half* of those who lose weight rapidly gain it back within 3 years, and 95% of the other half regain it in 5 years. Further, according to a recent survey by the Wheat Industry Council, about 28% of all Americans adhere to some weight-loss diet at any given time. And, incidentally, the 2.3 billion excess pounds that they carry, if converted from fat into gasoline, could run 900,000 automobiles for a year.

So, how do you defy such convincing statistics? By setting and striving for the equilibrium between eating and exercising that will stop the yo-yo at precisely the point you want it to remain. To achieve that equilibrium point, you must understand the value of exercise, whether you have bad knees, as Jody does, an aversion to sweating, as some people do, or a job, as plenty of people do, "that just doesn't afford me the time or opportunity to work out."

Whatever your present self-image, whether you consider yourself fat or fit, you probably want to achieve a long-term ideal weight for many reasons: vitality for your work and leisure activities, heightened self-esteem, a sense of physical and mental well-being, and the respect of others. Add sound medical reasons to your list, too.

Although the medical and physiological communities cannot yet isolate all the precise causes of obesity, all health professionals do agree on the tremendous health risks it poses and on its side effects, among them heart problems due to an overworked cardiac system, high blood pressure (hypertension), diabetes, gallbladder disease, high cholesterol levels, cancers (especially endometrial cancer), osteoarthritis and degenerative joint disease, and lung and kidney diseases.

The results of the Framingham Heart Study support the point. After a 26-year investigation, the researchers found that the chances of death increase 2 percent for each pound over the ideal weight. That means that a person 10 pounds overweight can expect a 20-percent increase in the odds of dying within 26 years. Before we explore the caloric value of exercises and see how Jody used them to regain her "fighting" weight, we need to understand just how metabolism turns calorie intake into calorie output.

HOW THE BODY TURNS FOOD INTO ENERGY OR FAT

One of the smallest components of human body cells are the mitochondria, tiny energy factories. These mitochondria use oxygen to transform food into energy, a process called metabolism.

It all starts at the mouth. You breathe in air with its high concentration of oxygen, and your lungs collect the oxygen in millions of small sacs called alveoli. The sacs empty their oxygen into surrounding tiny blood vessels known as capillaries by partial pressure diffusion.

The blood inside the capillaries carries particles known as red blood corpuscles, which contain hemoglobin, an iron-containing molecule that attaches itself to oxygen. The heart pumps the red blood corpuscles with their oxygen-laden hemoglobin through hundreds of miles of blood vessels to the living cells that need it for metabolism. Hence, an exercising body processes more oxygen than a sedentary one. Over time, as a person becomes more fit, his or her ability to process oxygen increases; this is the key to what it means to be aerobically fit. Smoking works against our oxygen-processing ability, but I won't pause here for my sermon on tar and nicotine.

The fit body also manufactures more hemoglobin than the unfit body, thus facilitating the collection of plenty of oxygen for the metabolic process, and it also develops hundreds more yards of microscopic vessels to carry oxygen to the mitochondria.

When the oxygen arrives at the cell level, close to the mitochondria, it joins the dietary fuel that has traveled from the mouth down the esophagus to the stomach, where the digestive system continues to break down the food. The food then passes through the gastrointestinal valve for final digestion in the large and small intestines. After the body has reduced the food to its six constituents—proteins, fats, carbohydrates, vitamins, minerals, and water—it transports them via the bloodstream to different locations. Assimilation occurs after the final breakdown of carbohydrates into blood sugars (or glycogen), protein into amino acids, and fats into fatty acids and triglycerides.

The digestion, absorption, and assimilation of the various nutrients drawn from the three nutrient sources requires different amounts of energy, depending on how quickly the body can break them down into fat and sugar fuel for the mitochondria factories. Protein burns nearly 25 percent of its total calories in the digestive process, not only because it takes a lot of energy to digest protein, but also because it requires a good deal of energy to break up the complex molecules and restructure them into amino acids in the liver.

I learned about high-fat diets at any early age. When our parents wanted me and my brothers to learn about calorie "costs," they encouraged us to choose an animal-raising project: One brother chose a dog, another a horse, and the third chickens. I picked beef cattle. When my dad suggested I try a new cattle feed mixed with fatty soybean oil, I quickly found my shorthorn steers gaining fat weight faster than they did without the oil added to the grain. The lesson? Body fat is similar to the fat in the foods we eat. The fat that we store comes in large part from the fat we eat.

Most dieters know that they should avoid high-fat diets, but few realize that high-protein weight-reduction diets can also cause problems. Many high-protein foods also contain a high percentage of fat (therefore more calories), and the body stores these fat calories very easily. Furthermore, the digestion of protein puts a good deal of strain on the liver and kidneys.

On the other hand, very little body fat comes from carbohydrates. Dr. Elliot Dansworth, a professor of medicine and director of the Clinical Research Center, College of Medicine, University of Vermont, reports, "We simply can say that fat in your body comes predominantly from the fat you eat—it doesn't come from the carbohydrates you eat." When you eat carbohydrates, you stimulate more heat loss than when you eat an equal number of fat calories.

The fit person eating a 60%–25%–15% diet obtains from the breakdown of carbohydrates the proper percentage of glycogen needed to move the muscles; the correct dose of fatty acids and triglycerides from fat to support activity and metabolism; and the right amount of amino acids from protein to rebuild cells.

The unfit body, on the other hand, lacks the balanced intermediary biochemical pathways for efficient assimilation of nutrients. Fit people are much better at burning fat calories than unfit people because they have a developed intermediary metabolic system. Without the demands of exercise, the need for carbohydrates and fats declines to the point where many remaining calories continue floating through the bloodstream. These extra calories, whether from dietary carbohydrates or fat, are converted into fat.

The body stores such fat selectively, first laying it down like cement between bricks inside the muscle fibers as intramuscular fat, or marbling. It also accumulates on the outside of the muscles and organs. Such extramuscular or subcutaneous fat forms the bulges we associate with overweight bodies.

Since people with genetically different body types tend to collect fat in different places on the body, researchers have concluded that heredity seems to play a determining role in where an individual stores his or her fat. Generally, men tend to carry it around their waistlines, while women collect it around their thighs and hips. That's why overweight men take the shape of apples and overweight women look like pears. And here's where women like Jody suffer. Fat stored in the hips and thighs of pear-shaped women seems to be more stable and harder to get rid of than fat around the waistlines of apple-shaped men. On the other side of the coin, however, pear shapes outlive apple shapes. Men with waists bigger than their hips succumb most frequently to such ailments as heart disease and high blood pressure.

Once food and oxygen come together in the living cells, metabolism—the transformation of food into energy—occurs. However, while oxygen passes easily through the wall of an individual muscle cell, the more complex blood sugars can't. So the catalyst, insulin, opens a space between the molecules of the cell wall so that the blood-sugar particle can slip inside. Once there, the still-complex blood-sugar molecule in the energy production process breaks down. Imagine a wood stove (the energy factory) that requires small pieces of wood (a substance called adrenosine triphosphate or ATP) and cannot accept big logs (blood sugars).

By the same token, fat, stored inside a fat cell as a triglyceride —a combination of fatty acid and glycerol—can't pass through the cell wall either. To get fat out of storage, another catalyst, epinephrine, excites an enzyme to divide the triglyceride and allow it into the bloodstream in the form of fatty acids, which, once again, the body can turn into useful energy (ATP). Again, the big logs have been cut into smaller pieces that the energy factories can accept.

Finally, a calorie, either obtained from food or brought out of fat storage, arrives inside a working cell to meet a molecule of oxygen, another recent arrival after an equally long trip. Metabolism begins.

The mitochondria factories work like the cylinders in your car: Oxygen, mixed in the carburetor with gasoline, squirts into a chamber where a spark can ignite it. When the mixture explodes (combustion), the released energy forces the piston to move and, in turn, drive the mechanical levers that turn the car engine over. After combustion, leftover substances, the exhaust fumes (including carbon monoxide, a gas poisonous to humans), are pushed from the engine's system and eliminated into the air. Similarly, oxygen and ATP enter the mitochondrial chamber, where a "spark" from the body's electrical nervous system produces combustion. Energy has now been transformed from energy input to energy output.

As with a car engine, your body must remove the by-products

of combustion. In simple terms, you generate two kinds of metabolic exhaust: aerobic and anaerobic. Both forms of exhaust include water and carbon dioxide, but anaerobic exhaust includes such substances as lactic acid. Aerobic exercise, like good food, benefits the body because it helps you burn more stored fat when you work out and because it provides more enjoyment. During aerobic exercise, the body takes in more oxygen than it needs, thus making it possible for you to continue to move and talk simultaneously. Anaerobic exercise benefits the body less because during anaerobic exercise the body takes in *less* oxygen than it needs. If you are training to become a champion, you actually want limited doses of this type of exercise. Anaerobic exercise requires high-carbohydrate fuel, burns little fat, and causes a buildup of lactic-acid levels. Lactic acid actually works to shut your muscles down and causes muscle fatigue. The carbon dioxide produced by both forms of exercise finds its way into the bloodstream, back to the heart, and eventually to the lungs for disposal into the air.

At this point, the energy factories have done their job. Interestingly, if you don't use the mitochondria, you lose them, but if you do use them, stoking them up to full working capacity, you grow more of them. The more mitochondria you grow, the more calories you can burn. In fact, as you exercise, your body produces 50–60 percent more of these tiny energy factories, which also gain in size. Therefore, exercise makes you a better fat and sugar burner.

Despite the foregoing simplification of the complexities surrounding the conversion of food into energy or fat, you now possess the facts that can put the Equilibrium Plan to work for you. Most important, exercise affects every cell in your body. If you increase your activity, exercising becomes increasingly easier and calorie burning more effective for the following reasons:

- An increase in the size and number of mitochondria, resulting in an increased ability to burn fat fuel
- An increase, up to 80 percent, in the amount of oxygen delivered to the muscles, as well as in the amount of oxygen carried by red blood corpuscles
- An increase in heart weight and size, resulting in greater

stroke volume, with each heartbeat pushing out a greater
amount of blood
- A drop in the resting heart rate
- A lowering of blood pressure
- Improved breathing functions
- Reduced cholesterol levels
- Less body fat

Recent research concludes that exercise creates cleaner and
more flexible blood vessels. Just as your garden hose, left in the
sun too long, becomes hard and inflexible, so do your vessels if left
inactive and fed a bad diet. Inactivity leads to a thickening and
clogging of the vessel's interior walls, forcing blood through a
more constricted space. The result: high blood pressure and
hardening of the arteries (arteriosclerosis).

COUNTING YOUR IDLE-SPEED CALORIES

The first law of thermodynamics states that energy is neither
created nor destroyed but rather is transformed from one state
to another. Scientists call this the principle of the conservation of
energy.

The chemical energy locked inside food follows this scientific
rule. When we eat our food, our digestive systems release the
trapped chemical energy, transforming some of it into heat energy but conserving most of it as chemical energy the body can,
in turn, transform into mechanical or kinetic energy by the action of our muscles and active tissues. A third energy conversion,
called transport energy, transfers the chemicals and other substances from body cell to body cell.

Just as scientists use the bomb calorimeter described in Chapter 2 to determine the number of calories stored in food, they
employ a similar kind of measuring chamber, called the human
calorimeter, to measure the calories we expend (see following
illustration). It involves putting an exercising individual inside
the chamber and measuring increases in body temperature with
a water bag that lines the chamber's inner wall.

Although highly accurate, this technique does not lend itself
to practical application in the everyday world. But using this and

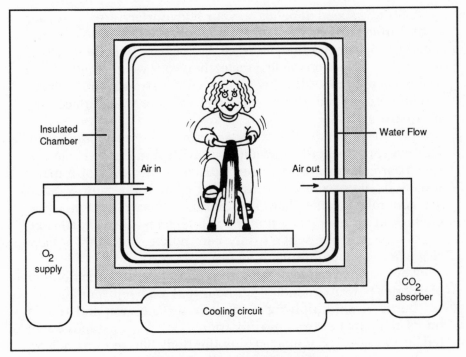

Insulated Chamber

Water Flow

Air in

Air out

O₂ supply

CO₂ absorber

Cooling circuit

The Human Calorimeter

other techniques, exercise physiologists can actually tell you how much of each of the three fuel sources—carbohydrates, fats, and protein—you burn while exercising. Thus, they can determine whether you are a fat burner or a carbohydrate burner, a distinction that will become very important to our discussion of exercise.

You may have seen a test in which a person walking or running on a treadmill breathes into a device that collects expired air. If you ever have a chance to take the test, do so without hesitation. It's painless, and it will put into your hands a powerful weapon in the war on weight. Meanwhile, though, you can easily calculate how many calories you expend in one day.

First, you must first know your resting metabolic rate, or idle speed, the minimum level of calories your body needs to sustain itself while at rest. You can calculate your own quite easily. All the math throughout this book is easy. Take some time now to compute your values.

Your idle speed depends on your body surface area, and your body surface area is derived from a combination of height and weight. Look at the Body Surface Area Chart *(following)*. First locate your height on the first scale, then your weight on the third scale. Then connect the two points with a straight line. Where the line crosses the second scale, you will find your surface area in square meters.

The larger your body surface area, the higher your idle speed. However, two other factors affect individual idle speed: age and sex. Your idle speed decreases with age, with that of females usually 5–10 percent lower than that of males because women are generally smaller than men and usually carry a higher percentage of fat *(see chart under Body Surface Area Chart)*. Fat, a less metabolically active tissue than muscle, burns fewer calories when the body remains at rest.

Now you can pinpoint your idle speed by taking the number of calories per square meter per hour that a person your age and sex burns and multiplying it by your surface area and the 24 hours in a day. For example, my friend Jack Taylor stands 6 feet tall and weighs 165 pounds. Using the Body Surface Area Chart, he determines a surface area of 1.98. Given his age (41) and his sex (male), he then uses the Age and Sex Chart of Metabolic Rates to pinpoint the calories per square meter that his body burns: 38. Multiplying the surface area by calories per square meter (1.98 × 38), he obtains 75.24 calories per square meter per hour. Finally, to arrive at his daily idle speed, he multiplies 75.24 by 24 hours to get his idle speed of 1,806 calories burned per day.

Using this method, I have calculated my own idle speed at 1,434 calories per day. In 1985, as part of an experiment on endurance triathletes, I underwent very sophisticated tests in the University of Pennsylvania's Environmental Physiology Department. The school's physiologists computed my idle speed at 1,422 calories, or within .008 of the accuracy of our method. Every activity beyond rest will add calories to my basic idle speed. Even if I do nothing but vegetate, I must consume 1,422 calories a day. In this light, it becomes rather frightening to realize that many of the fad diets on the market today recommend daily calorie intakes below their followers' idle speeds. On such diets, you would not consume enough even for a life of total inactivity.

Of course, none of us want to live like a vegetable, and we spend our days making our beds, brushing our teeth, walking to

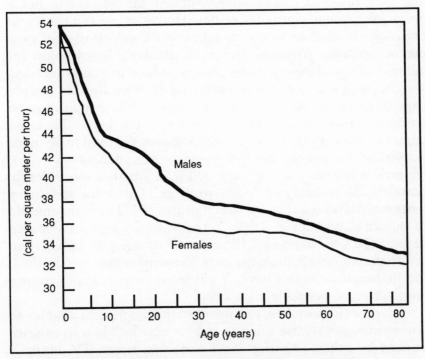

Body Surface Area Chart

Height Scale
(inches)

Surface Area Scale
(square meters)

Weight Scale
(lbs)

Age and Gender Chart of Metabolic Rates

(cal per square meter per hour)

Males

Females

Age (years)

work, rushing around to get ready for an important date, dancing at the local nightclub, and engaging in sexual activity. Your total daily caloric expenditure varies as your muscle-to-fat ratio varies (muscles burn 20 percent of your idling calories), as you move from climate to climate (adjusting to cold weather consumes calories), and as life's exigencies, from illnesses to pregnancies, take their caloric toll. Rather than getting bogged down in all the individual and environmental influences on the expenditure of calories in your daily life, you should just remember that your total expenditure includes idle-speed calories, job-related calories, and other calories burned by various activities. However, no one factor adds calories to the idle speed more than physical exercise.

COUNTING YOUR JOB, EXERCISE, AND OTHER CALORIES

In addition to your idle-speed calories, there are three other types of calories that you expend each day: those spent on the job, those spent exercising, and those burned by other daily activities. Job calories represent those that you expend at your occupation, and they resist easy calculation. Not only do jobs differ, but a given job can vary from day to day. However, we can use some textbook calculations to gain insight into the calorie costs of various occupations. Although the work situations listed below involve decreasing expenditures, you must bear in mind that body weight plays a major role in each case because heavier people expend more calories than lighter people while doing the same work—it takes more energy to move a big body the same amount. Age is a player in the calorie game. We tend to be more active and burn more calories when we are younger.

Jack works as a writer and editor, a job that most closely parallels the category of "office workers." Given the sedentary nature of his occupation, he would probably fall near the middle of the scale, perhaps at 2,520. Actually, as we'll see in a couple of pages, Jack burns about 3,122 calories per day *with* his exercise program, but only 2,402 without it. Remember that we are dealing in rough estimates here. We'll learn how to figure calorie costs far more precisely a bit later.

Given its importance, I've devoted the whole next chapter to a discussion of exercise calories, but for now let's look at calories burned by other activities. Next time you watch TV, observe

TOTAL CALORIES BURNED PER DAY BY OCCUPATION

Occupation	Minimum	Maximum	Average
Forestry workers	2,860	4,600	3,670
Coal miners	2,970	4,560	3,660
Farmers	2,450	4,670	3,550
University students	2,270	4,440	2,930
Laboratory technicians	2,240	3,820	2,840
Office workers	1,820	3,820	2,520
Retail Clerks	1,820	2,850	2,250
Houseworkers	1,760	2,320	2,090

which of your fellow viewers moves the most during the commercials. Invariably, the leaner watchers hop up and scurry around, trying to get something done before the program begins again. Exercise experts call such calorie expenditures nonsensible, not because they don't make sense but because they represent all the extra energy that slimmer people invest in numerous little tasks. The slim people don't even realize they are burning energy that their more fat-laden friends usually label senseless.

Indeed, for really obese people, simply hoisting themselves out of a TV recliner and waddling to the refrigerator for another calorie binge can become an anaerobic activity as their heart rates shoot up and they find themselves breathing hard. In addition, with even light exercise, they burn a high percentage of carbohydrate calories because their muscles must move such large masses. Meanwhile, their skinnier counterparts burn a higher percentage of fat fuel performing the same task. Try another experiment. In a roomful of friends, ask the group to help fetch something. Invariably the leanest one volunteers. Skinnier people enjoy expending nonsensible calories.

It's difficult to calculate precisely the expenditure of these other calories because few people consciously plan to spend them. However, in Chapter 6 you will see how you can make these types of caloric expenditures a more conscious part of your daily Equilibrium Plan. When most people visualize a workout, they picture a jog in the park, an aerobic dance class, or a Nautilus machine, but I will show you how your shower, gardening tools, vacuum cleaner, and even your office desk can become effective workout machines.

To compute the calories you burn in daily activities, consult the following table, which lists the total or gross calories, including idle speed, burned by each activity. If you can't find the exact activity, use one that seems to involve a similar level of strenuousness. Look under the weight category that you currently maintain (remember, you burn more calories if you are heavier) and read the number of calories burned per half hour of the activity.

GROSS CALORIES BURNED PER HALF HOUR IN DAILY ACTIVITIES

	BODY WEIGHT					
Activity	110	130	150	170	190	210
Sitting; talking	39	45	51	57	66	72
Cooking dinner	51	60	69	78	87	96
Lawn mowing	168	198	228	258	288	318
Piano playing	60	72	81	93	102	114
Typing	42	48	54	60	69	78
Washing dishes (hand)	54	60	66	72	78	84

Next, multiply the number of calories burned per half hour for your weight category by the number of half hours you invest in this activity each day. Let's suppose that Jack spends his 24 hours per day sleeping 8 hours and working 8 hours (as an editor, he burns 66 calories per half hour × 16 for a total of 1056). That leaves him with 8 hours of "free" time, which he spends as follows:

Activity	Calories per Half Hour	Time Spent (half hours)	Total Calories
Driving to and from work each day	48	4	192
Sitting and eating four meals	48	4	192
Working out (swims crawl fast)	360	2	720
Writing	66	2	132
Watching TV	48	2	96
Talking on phone	57	1	57
Ironing	75	1	75
		8 hours	1,464 calories

If Jack subtracts the exercise portion (720 swimming calories), he finds that he nets 744 other calories per day in various "free-time" activities as part of his daily life-style.

Perhaps you can control your job or other activities in such a way that they will help you achieve your ideal level of total exercise calories, but if you are like most of us in this office-oriented information society, you must set up a deliberate exercise plan to get there.

Calories burned from working out will become your most powerful weapon in your struggle to reach and maintain your ideal weight. For every minute that you vigorously exercise, you burn several times more calories than at your resting rate. While my normal metabolic rate burns about 1 calorie per minute, my typical run consumes 13 calories per minute. Now that's one quick way to increase the burning of calories!

The following table displays the numbers of calories burned by several of the most common and popular forms of exercise. I have arranged them with the ones that burn the most calories per minute at the top. This doesn't mean that you should value the top ones more than the bottom ones, because you should allow for the intensity of any given exercise. The harder you exercise, the more calories you burn. For example, cycling for an hour at 20 miles per hour burns more calories than cycling for an hour at 10 miles per hour. Be sure to take your body weight into account, because the more weight you carry over a certain distance, the more calories you burn.

GROSS CALORIES BURNED PER HALF HOUR DURING TYPICAL EXERCISES

Exercise Activity	WEIGHT					
	110	130	150	170	190	220
Running, 8 mph	312	357	402	447	492	537
Basketball (full court)	294	336	378	420	462	504
Cycling, 10 mph	258	294	330	366	402	438
Football (touch)	234	267	303	336	369	402
Tennis	168	189	213	237	255	276
Walking, 3 mph	117	135	153	171	189	207
Swimming, 20 yards per min	117	135	153	171	189	207
Golf (cart)	87	99	111	123	135	147

You now possess the knowledge you need to determine the calories on the exercise side of your fitness equation. Let's see how Jack does it. We have already calculated from the Body Surface Area Chart that he idles at 1,806 calories per day. But since the calories expended in Jack's other activities are gross calories (i.e., the calculations *include* idle-speed calories), we only list the time Jack spends actually sleeping under idle speed. Thus, Jack's total daily calorie expenditure is as follows:

Job calories 1,056
Exercise calories 720
Other calories 744
Idle speed (sleep) . . . 602 (1,806 divided by 3 = 8 hours sleep)
  Total calories 3,122

What do these numbers tell Jack? First and foremost, if he cut out his exercise program, he would drop down to 2,402 calories, about average for an adult man. But 1 hour of workout per day accounts for 23 percent of his total calories, which is more than half as many as the job calories he expends during his 8 hours at the office. More important, he also avoids filling his fat cells and ballooning out.

Of course, no one wants to wear an oxygen-capturing mask or become a human calculator in order to compute calories burned. But the exercise calories side of the Equilibrium Plan Slide Guide described later on in this chapter, will help you with these calculations.

ESTIMATING YOUR BODY-FAT PERCENTAGE

The calories you expend through exercise depend on your total body weight, which is the sum of your lean body weight plus the weight of your fat. Life insurance companies define excess weight in terms of a height/weight chart, but height and weight only tell part of the story. Since your total weight consists of fat weight and muscle-essential weight, my Equilibrium Plan definition includes that important fat weight.

I say you are "overfat" if you carry 5 percent more than the scientifically accepted desirable body fat levels, which is 15 percent or less of the total weight for men and 25 percent or less for women. In other words, an overfat man's body exceeds 20 percent fat, while an overfat woman's exceeds 30 percent fat. Thus, if you are a 150-pound woman of average height with 45 pounds of fat weight, you are overfat, and if you are a 195-pound man of average height with 40 pounds of fat weight, you, too, are overfat.

The most accurate determination of your own body fat percentage involves underwater, or hydrostatic, weighing. Other methods include skin impedance (electrodes connecting the body to a computer), skin-fold calculations (measuring the thickness of pinched skin), and determination of body-part circumference (anthropometric measurements).

"Fat floats; muscle sinks." Go to any swimming pool and watch the fat-full bodies bouncing on top of the water and the lean, muscular, fat-low bodies working hard to stay afloat. Of the four popular tests, underwater weighing provides the most accurate method of measuring fat percentage, but since it requires expensive testing equipment, I will teach you the anthropometric approach. However, if you ever have an opportunity to be hydrostatically weighed, do so, because the results will sharpen the accuracy of the measurement of your fat-to-lean ratio.

To obtain a rough but still useful fat-to-lean ratio for yourself, you need only a measuring tape and the Body Fat Percent Charts (following). If you are a man, measure your waistline exactly at the level of your navel. Be careful not to let the tape slip up or down, and keep the pressure firm, not restrictive. Next, with a ruler, line up your waist circumference or waist girth with your pounds of body weight on the following chart. Note where the ruler crosses the "Body Fat %" line on the chart. That tells you your current fat level. The dotted line shows the percent fat for a 170-pound man whose waist measures 34 inches.

If you are a woman, measure the circumference around your hips at their widest point. To find the percent fat, connect the circumference of your hips and your height (not your body weight) on the following chart. Where the line crosses the "Body Fat" line you will find your percent body fat.

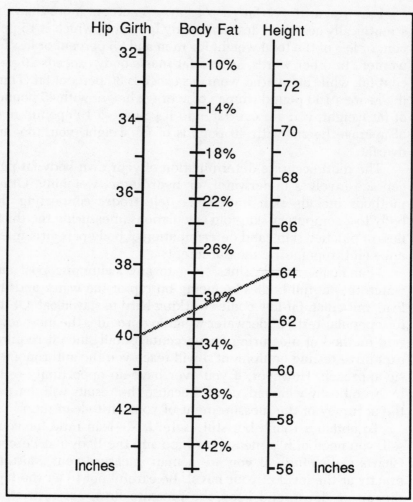

Body Fat Percent Chart for Women

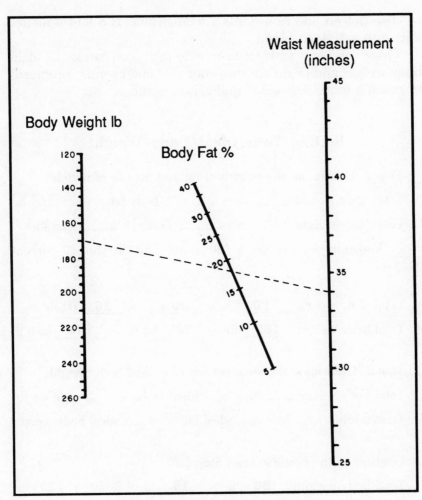

Body Fat Percent Chart for Men

The dotted line represents a woman who is 5 feet 4 inches tall, with a 40-inch hipline.

Once you know your fat-to-muscle ratio, you can set an ideal body weight and begin altering your diet and exercise programs to reach a more desirable equilibrium point.

Setting Your Ideal Body Weight

Step 1. Determine the pounds of fat and pounds of muscle:

A. Total body weight _____ lb × _____% body fat = _____ fat lb

B. Total body weight _____ lb − _____ fat lb = _____ lean lb

For example, consider a 180-pound man carrying 20 percent body fat:

A. Total body weight __180__ lb × __20%__ = __36__ fat lb

B. Total body weight __180__ lb − __36__ fat lb = __144__ lean lb

Step 2. Determine the ideal pounds of fat and body weight:

C. Total body weight ____ lb × ____ ideal % fat = ____ ideal fat lb

D. Lean pounds ____ lb + ____ ideal fat lb = ____ ideal body weight

Continuing the example from Step 1:

C. Total body weight __180__ lb × __15__ ideal % fat = __27__ ideal fat lb

D. Lean pounds __144__ lb + __27__ ideal fat lb = __171__ ideal body weight.

Although a bit rough, these calculations will give you a clear enough idea of your fat-to-lean ratio to proceed with a consideration of how exercise affects weight control. It might surprise you to learn that your best body weight is quite close to how much you weighed at the age of 20.

A final word about computing percent of body fat. Some types of people defy the averages. If you are extremely fat or skinny, or if you play serious competitive sports, you should invest in an underwater testing session.

EXERCISE AND WEIGHT CONTROL

Carrying a fat-full body through an exercise workout is, in many ways, like carrying an extra person on your back. Imagine having to run with a 20- or 30-pound child in your arms. That child weighs and slows you down, but it also increases your workload and consequently the number of calories that you expend.

If you run at 10 mph, you burn twice the number of calories *per hour* than if you run at 5 mph. If you run the *same distance,* you burn the same number of calories no matter what your speed. At 5 mph you would run 1 mile in 12 minutes, while at 10 mph you would finish the same mile in 6 minutes. The same holds true for marathoners. If you weigh 137 pounds and run the 26-mile race in 2 hours, you expend 2,600 calories; if you run it in 4 hours, you still burn the same number of calories as the speedster. However, the overweight marathoner carrying excess poundage over the 26-mile course will burn a good deal more calories than the slimmer runners.

Physiologists using an obesity classification that measures the number and size of fat cells have discovered two kinds of fatness: one involving larger fat cells (hypertrophy) and one involving a greater number of fat cells (hyperplasia). In clinical studies comparing overweight and fit people, in which the overweight groups averaged 35 percent more fat in each fat cell than the fit, scientists discovered that the total number of fat cells in the overfat person averaged *three times* the number found in the fit. In one of the most widely respected studies, from the University of Massachusetts, the overweight had 75 billion fat cells, compared to 27 billion for their lean counterparts. In extreme cases of obesity, fat cell counts have exceeded 260 billion!

The average fat person studied displayed a cell size of 0.6 (measured as micrograms lipid per cell), and obese people showed a 0.9 cell size; but since the number of fat cells totaled 26 cells per billion versus 77 per billion, the number of cells clearly outranked size as the critical factor in obesity.

Another important fact also came to light when research revealed that after weight loss the number of cells remained the same, indicating that as you lose fat weight, you simply shrink cell size, not number.

This explains why overweight people who have lost weight from a diet-only regimen despair of ever keeping the fat weight off. Fat cells cannot get out of your body; you can only fill them up or empty them out.

However, studies of individuals with no history of obesity who had been forced to double their fat intake from 14 to 28 percent showed no increase in the number of fat cells. When these fattened volunteers returned to their former skinny selves, sure enough, researchers found the same number of fat cells as at the beginning of the experiment. This means that if you eat more calories than you burn, you fill your existing fat cells without adding new ones.

There may be periods in adulthood when fat cells might start multiplying in number, but researchers have not yet pinpointed them. However, they know that fat cells do increase in number during three specific phases of childhood: (1) the latter part of infancy (0–3 years), (2) the time of starting school (5–6 years), and (3) adolescence (12–18 years).

It would seem that childhood obesity involves increasing the number of fat cells, while adult obesity generally involves creating only *larger* cells. Parents should pay particular attention to these facts, stressing proper exercise and eating habits for their kids. Childhood or adolescent obesity clearly sets you up for fat adulthood by giving you so many more fat cells to fill. If fat kids fail on the playground, they may avoid playing, thus missing a key opportunity to eliminate excess calories throughout their lives. Inactivity causes the rapid onset of obesity, not to mention destruction of self-image. And a negative self-image, established during adolescence, persists into adulthood.

In addition to the number and size of the fat cells in your body, other factors are at work that affect your ability to lose weight. Recent scientific research indicates that the hypothalamus, a coordinating center located at the base of the brain, controls two vital body functions: temperature and weight. It triggers such temperature mechanisms as shivering and sweating, and it supervises fat regulation. The hypothalamus also lowers

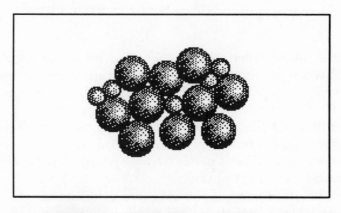

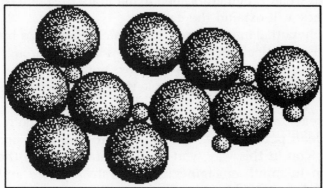

Dieting Changes the Size, Not the Number of Fat Cells

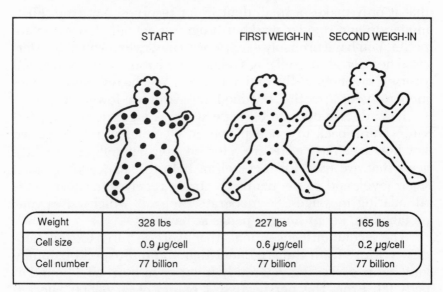

	START	FIRST WEIGH-IN	SECOND WEIGH-IN
Weight	328 lbs	227 lbs	165 lbs
Cell size	0.9 μg/cell	0.6 μg/cell	0.2 μg/cell
Cell number	77 billion	77 billion	77 billion

Changes in Fat Cells with Weight Loss

your idle speed when you restrict your intake of calories and raises it when you increase your intake, in an attempt to maintain your weight at a point of equilibrium. In a related maneuver, the amount of a certain chemical that helps the body store fat increases dramatically when calorie intake is reduced. This means that when you eat fewer calories, your body fights you, trying to store them as fat. That's partly why fat people stay fat, by working against their own physiology.

On the other hand, if you eat more calories than your hypothalamus weight regulators need to maintain the point of equilibrium, they will expend the calories.

The hypothalamus triggers a chemical that helps burn calories. This chemical encourages millions of cells throughout the body to burn off extra energy calories. Not surprisingly, we find more of it in normal-weight people than in overweight individuals.

To reach a new equilibrium point with lower body fat and higher lean percentages, and to prevent your own body from fighting you in this way, you must constantly keep the fitness equation in mind, engaging in moderate exercise and eating good foods/good calories.

Most fad diets promote two falsehoods, claiming that exercise causes an increase in appetite and that it burns so few calories that it only makes a small dent in fat reserves. Not true. First, moderate and regular workout programs actually lower the appetite. You have probably experienced days when you have exercised heavily, as in a full day's hiking in the mountains, and found yourself ravenous at the end of the day. Yes, heavy exercise does increase your appetite, but moderate exercise lowers it.

How does moderate exercise work as an appetite suppressant? Think back to our explanation of metabolism, where we saw how free fatty acids are released from fat cells. These fatty acids that are used for metabolism help to balance your blood sugar level, and consequently the brain receives fewer hunger-stimulating messages. So moderate exercise, which raises your metabolism, keeps hunger pangs at bay.

The second misconception—that exercise burns too few calories—springs from the argument that you must spend painfully long hours exercising vigorously in order to burn off a pound of body fat. From this perspective, 1 pound of fat (3,500 calories) equals 10 hours of golf or 5 hours of aerobics. True. However, if you played those 10 hours of golf 2 hours per day twice a week, you would lose that pound in 2½ weeks. That's not bad, when you picture a pound of butter no longer spread around your midriff.

Whenever your intake falls below your output, you shed body weight. But exactly what kind of weight do you lose? If you maintain a basically sedentary life-style, the first weight loss measured on the bathroom scale usually reflects water and carbohydrate reduction. With further dietary restriction but no workout, you will lose fat from within the fat cells, as well as valuable muscle. If, however, you combine a dietary program with a workout program, you increase fat burning and as long as your workload is moderate you don't lose muscle; you get stronger and more energetic.

If you require 1,500 calories and you decrease your caloric input to a 1,000-calorie-a-day carbohydrate diet combined with 2½ hours of moderate exercise each day, your body will go through three phases. During the first 3 days you will lose 70 percent water and 25 percent fat. By day 11 through 13, you will mostly lose fat and a little water, until day 21, when you will lose 85 percent fat and no water. The chart, What You Really Lose, clearly shows that since the body protects its fat by expelling water first, losing fat weight requires some patience.

The body's reluctance to shed fat first explains why diets alone only give the illusion of success, and it argues for a sustained commitment to the Equilibrium Plan. In addition, dieting alone results in decreased muscle size. Just as unused fat cells lose dimension, so, too, do unused muscle cells. However, while low-calorie diets, especially those that prescribe low protein, break down muscle fiber to make their calories available for fuel, you need that muscle tissue to maintain your energy level. Ironically, then, just when you most desperately need active muscle to burn more calories, you lose it if you try to lose weight only by dieting.

THE EXERCISE SIDE OF THE SLIDE GUIDE

On the exercise side of the Slide Guide, you will find all four parts of the exercise half of the fitness equation. First, you will see the

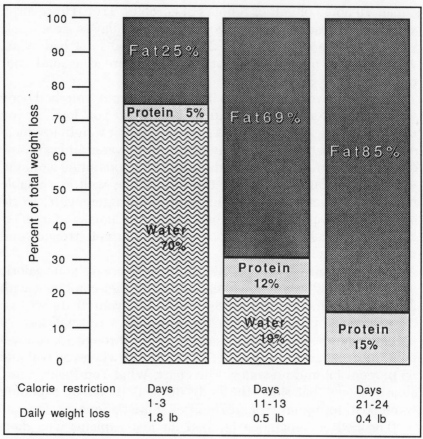

What You Really Lose: Water, Protein, and Fat

three activities you can control: job calories, exercise calories, and other calories. The fourth part shows idle speeds for every 20 pounds of weight carried by both women and men.

Since the more your body weighs, the more calories you will expend in a given activity, the exercise side of the Slide Guide lets you tailor the numbers to your own particular weight.

The use of the exercise side of the Slide Guide involves five steps:

1. Select your activity heading (Job, Exercise, or Other).
2. Put your current body weight in the window next to your selection.

3. Find the specific activity in question.
4. Read the number of calories burned per half hour.
5. Multiply the half hour figure by the number of half hours you perform the activity.

For example, in the morning, I run an hour at a pace of 1 mile per 7 minutes. To count the number of calories I expend during this run, I select "Exercise Calories," moving the number 130 (the closest value to my 125-pound body weight) into the window, then read below it to find "Running—8 mph" The window shows 357 calories per half hour, so I multiply 357 by 2 to obtain a total of 714 calories burned per hour running.

Since I also like to bike an hour after work, I would add an hour on the bike averaging 10 mph. Looking under "Exercise Calories" and finding "Bicycling, 10 mph," I can check at the window to see that bicycling burns 294 calories per half hour. I multiply 294 by 2, for a total of 588 calories for an hour of cycling.

On a typical day, I spend 9 hours at the office, mostly in meetings or working with my franchisees. To determine job calories, I place the 130 in the window for my weight and find under the heading "Managerial (active)" that I burn 2,052 calories on the job (18 half hours × 114 = 2,052).

What about other daily activities? I spend the 6 "free" hours left in my day as follows: 1 hour housework (cleaning at 111 calories per half hour), 1 hour reading (sitting at 45 per half hour), 1 hour eating (42 per half hour), 2 hours typing (48 per half hour), a half hour grooming (taking a shower, brushing my teeth, etc., at 90 per half hour), and 30 minutes commuting to and from work (42 per half hour).

Putting all this together, I multiply the number of half hours spent on each of the activities by the number of calories burned per half hour to obtain a grand total of 694 other calories burned.

I usually sleep 8 hours a night. Sleeping burns calories at my idle speed times the number of hours I sleep. Earlier in this chapter we calculated my idle speed at 0.98 calorie per minute (or 29.4 per half hour), so 29.4 multiplied by 16 results in 470 calories burned sleeping. Now, let's tally my full caloric expenditure for a typical day:

Job Calories 2,052
Exercise calories
    Running 714
    Bicycling 588
Other calories 694
Sleeping (idle speed) calories 470
    Total calories burned: 4,518

Despite my sedentary job, I burn quite a few calories each day with habitual exercise. In fact, I burn almost 35 percent of my calories with planned workouts, nearly as much as I burn during 9 hours at work and even more than some people burn during 24 hours at their idle speeds.

YOUR PERSONAL EXERCISE CALORIES LOG

Now you can use your Slide Guide to fill out your own Exercise Calories Log, to see how it stacks up against the figures in the Diet Calories Log you filled in earlier. That's what my friend Jody Carper did. Finally deciding to conquer her weight problem once and for all, Jody performed the calculations I've been recommending in this chapter.

In Jody's case, she will eventually compare her total output to her total intake, combining them into a balanced plan for lifetime fitness, but these calculations alone convinced her to get started by adding some exercise to her daily expenditure. She stopped using her bad knees as an excuse not to exercise and started working out regularly.

When I saw her 6 months later, I could hardly believe my eyes: She not only went down to 165 pounds, she looked fit and energetic. Seeing the delight in my eyes, she summed up her success in one sentence, "Sally, I quit dieting and bought a dog." A dog? "We walk together an hour every day at his pace. It has changed my life and, as you can see, my body. All those years and over fifty different diets and I just kept gaining weight. You were right. But it took a schnauzer."

I had my dogs with me at the time, so I knew their value as workout machines. Her long walks with Clover increased Jody's idle speed and created an entire life-style shift for her.

EXERCISE CALORIES LOG

NAME: _____ **Jody Carper** _____   DATE: _____ **September 30, 1986** _____

Height: _____ **5'9"** _____   Weight: _____ **200 lb** _____   Age: _____ **38 years** _____

Body surface area: _____ **2.05 square meters** _____

Idle speed: **2.05 square meters × 36 calories per square meter per hour × 24 hours = 1,771.2 calories per day.** (To calculate your idle speed during sleep, multiply the figure for square meters times calories per square meter per hour times the number of hours you sleep per day.)

Total calorie expenditure per day:

Job:	**1,344**
Exercise:	**0**
Other activities:	**1,056**
Idle speed (sleep):	**590** **(8 hours 1,771 ÷ 3)**
Total:	**2,980** calories

Percent body fat: **34**

Pounds of fat: **68**

Lean pounds: **132**

Ideal percent body fat: **25**

Ideal body weight: **165**

Your own creative exercise program can do the same for you.

Jody walked off 35 pounds this way. Though her bad knees wouldn't let her run, they actually grew stronger with the walking. Not only does she find walking easy and fun, but it has created a wonderful bond with her pet.

Over time Jody's exercise increased her muscle weight and added active muscle tissue that burns more calories and decreases fat percent. With her new 25 percent fat/75 percent lean body, Jody felt better, looked better, and began enjoying life and work more. Believe it or not, without all that excess weight on them, her knees improved so much that she decided to take up a mild jogging program. But her little schnauzer is a walker, not a runner, so Jody has bought a 50-pound golden retriever. Now she walks with Clover and runs with Holly.

EXERCISE CALORIES LOG

NAME: _____ DATE: _____

Height: _____ Weight: _____ Age: _____

Body surface area: _____ square meters

Idle speed: _____ square meters × _____ calories per square
meter per hour × 24 hours = _____ calories per day. (To
calculate your idle speed during sleep, multiply the figure for
square meters times calories per square meter per hour times
the number of hours you sleep per day.)

Total calorie expenditure per day: Job: _____

Exercise: _____

Other activities: _____

Idle speed (sleep):   _____

Total: _____ calories

Percent body fat: _____

Pounds of fat: _____

Lean pounds: _____

Ideal percent body fat: _____

Ideal body weight: _____

CHAPTER 4

EQUILIBRIUM

BALANCE FOR LIFE

I have talked about the diet merry-go-round and the yo-yo phenomenon, which cause perennial dieters who don't exercise to find their weight going up and down as they move from one fad approach to another. I also showed how Jack Taylor, a relatively fit 40-year-old man, and Jody Carper, a severely overweight 38-year-old woman, started their Equilibrium Plans. Jack began by watching what he ate more closely, while Jody paid more attention to daily exercise. Of course, to reach their ideal weights and stay there, they needed to control both sides of the fitness equation, much the way Sharon Barboni did.

Sharon is 26 years old, a secretary at a large electronics firm, and 28 pounds above her ideal weight. When she started the Equilibrium Plan, she chose as her ideal representation a portrait of herself as her high school's homecoming queen: a 5-foot 2-inch, 115-pound dark-haired beauty who had captained her school's soccer team. She had begun to see the pointer on her bathroom scale creeping higher and higher about 2 years after graduation from the local community college, and 6 months after her marriage to her childhood sweetheart, Steve Barboni. Without spring and fall soccer training and summer lifeguarding to burn off calories, and eating more than ever as she cooked large meals for herself and her husband, Sharon found herself adding about 5 pounds of fat tissue per year. Finally, after 5 years of disequilibrium, she tipped the scales at 143 pounds, and even Steve began urging her to go on a diet.

Like so many weight-conscious individuals, Sharon selected a starvation-diet plan first, cutting her calorie intake to half her idle-speed requirements. Sitting at her desk each day, she would listen to her stomach growling, and though she had begun swimming several laps each noon rather than eating lunch, she quickly found her energy level too low to continue the workout. Oh, she dropped 12 pounds, but a week after buying a sexy new dress for her sixth wedding anniversary celebration (which included dinner at the best steak house in town), she found that a lot of that fat had returned. The diet fell by the wayside, and 6 weeks later she almost cried when she weighed herself and saw the pointer indicating 148 pounds.

A friend then persuaded her that she should exercise off all that unwanted weight, so Sharon leaped into an arduous workout program with all the enthusiasm with which she had recently starved herself. If she could exercise off ten times more calories than usual and if she cut her food intake in half, she figured she could get down to 120 pounds overnight. Unfortunately, this strategy backfired, too. Convinced that she could not afford a minute of idleness, she whirled through a blur of activity, lifting weights, jogging, playing tennis, and swimming. After 3 days her body ached all over, and the recurrence of an old soccer injury to her back forced her off the program altogether. The result: no gain in her war on weight, but plenty of pain.

Twice Sharon had failed to achieve lasting results. Then she really tried balancing her fitness equation. She changed her habits, setting in motion long-term shifts in behavior that permanently reset her equilibrium point. On the diet side she recorded all the information on what and how much she ate. She recorded her input calories for 3 random days using the Diet Calories Log on page 50, and discovered she was averaging 2,400 calories per day from her diet. She cut back 500 in calories per day and embarked on a 1,900-calorie-per-day diet plan.

On the exercise side, Sharon added 500 calories per day of output activities by riding her bike to work, walking on her lunch hour, and taking 5-minute exercise breaks rather than coffee breaks. She also decided to exercise while watching her favorite evening television program.

Read through Sharon's Diet Calories Log and her Exercise Calories Log and you will see how she managed to burn 500 calories more and to eat 500 calories less per day for a 1,000-calorie-per-day deficit. Remember that over 7 days, those 7,000 calories represent 2 pounds of fat loss—with no muscle shrinkage.

Sharon eats three meals and snacks on a typical day like the one she noted on October 2, for a total of 1,886 calories. On the other side of the equation, she burns 2,931 calories. Total deficit: 1,045 calories.

Over the years I have competed in many arenas, from business to ultra-athletics, and I have fought to get the most out of every aspect of my personal and professional life. Whenever I have achieved any measure of success in my endeavors, I have done so by adhering to one simple rule: the principle of equilibrium. Most successful people I know offset work with play, personal satisfaction with social contributions, and material success with emotional or spiritual fulfillment. All those who succeed at lifelong fitness balance the fitness equation.

You've probably watched your own weight seesaw around a certain number on your bathroom scale, but if you want to stop the pointer at one number and keep it there for the rest of your life, you need only follow two fundamental rules of balance:

RULE 1: When diet calories = exercise calories, your body weight will remain constant. You will have achieved equilibrium.

RULE 2: When exercise calories exceed diet calories, your body weight will decrease. Conversely, when diet calories exceed exercise calories, your body weight will increase.

If you do not wish to alter your current weight, you can follow Rule 1, maintaining your present state of equilibrium. If you wish to take weight off and keep it off, you can follow Rule 2 until you

DIET CALORIES LOG

NAME: Sharon Barboni   DATE: October 2, 1986

	Code	Serving Size	Calories	Number of Servings	Calories
Meal					
Bran flakes cereal	○	1 1/3 cups	180	1	180
Skim milk	○	1 cup	86	1	86
Whole-wheat bread	○	1 slice	65	1	65
Banana	○	1 piece	105	1	105
Glass of water	○	1 cup	0	1	0
Total meal calories 436					
Meal					
Yogurt, nonfat, plain	○	1 cup	90	1	90
Bagel, 3 ounces	○	1	255	1	255
Fruit soda	○	12 oz	156	1	156
Total meal calories 501					
Meal					
Frozen entree: zucchini lasagna, vegetarian	○	4 ounces	260	1	260
Skim milk	○	1 cup	86	1	86
Lettuce	○	1 cup	6.8	3	20
Tomato	○	1 medium	25	1	25
Low-fat dressing	○	1 Tbs	15.8	2	31
Whole-wheat bread	○	1 slice	65	1	65
Applesauce	○	½ cup	53	2	106
Total meal calories 593					
Snacks					
Orange	○	1 piece	62	1	62
Apple, 5 ounces	○	1 piece	81	1	81
Pear, 5 ounces	○	1 piece	98	1	98
Popcorn, plain	○	1 cup	23	5	115
Total snack calories 356					
Total calories for day: 1,886					

reach your desired weight, then observe Rule 1 to remain at your new equilibrium point.

Sharon needs to practice Rule 2 because, like so many of us, she suffers from creeping obesity, the tendency to gain fat weight with age. Most of us begin experiencing this problem about age 25, as the body slowly adds 1 or 2 pounds of fat and drops the same amount of lean muscle each year. The phenomenon usually is the result of creeping sedentaryism—increased inactivity coupled with higher levels of caloric intake.

EXERCISE CALORIES LOG

NAME: _____**Sharon Barboni**_____ DATE: _____**October 2, 1986**_____

Height: _____**5'2"**_____ Weight: _____**143 pounds**_____ Age: _____**26**_____

Idle speed: __**1.66**__ square meters $\times$ __**36**__ calories per square meter $\times$ 24 hours = __**1,434**__ calories per day

Total calorie expenditure per day:

Job: __**1,104 (69 calories burned per half hour as a secretary times**__ $\times$ __**16 half hours)**__ + __**203 (50 from two 5-minute exercise breaks plus 153 from walking 1/2 hour at lunch time)**__ = __**1,307**__

Exercise: __**330 (two 15-minute bike rides, to and from work)**__

Other: __**816 (working in home, watching TV, at 51 calories per half hour**__ $\times$ __**16)**__

Idle speed (sleep): __**1,434**__ (from above) $\times$ __**.33**__ (8 hours, one-third of the day) = __**478**__

Total: __**2,931 calories**__

Percent body fat: __**32**__

Pounds of fat: __**46**__

Lean pounds: __**97**__

Ideal percent body fat: __**25**__

Ideal body weight: __**115**__

As we grow older, our combination of job, exercise, idle, and other calories may fall below the number of calories we eat. By the age of 35, an annual loss of muscle tissue and an annual gain of 1–2 pounds of fat weight may result in 10–20 pounds of excess baggage around the midsection, thighs, or hips.

It can even happen to a professional athlete. Throughout college I lived an unusually active life, participating in competitive sports and eating whatever I wanted, but when I went to Vietnam, I began exercising less and eating more. Long Binh, Da Nang, and Cam Ranh Bay lacked the playing fields and gymnasiums of the University of California, so I gradually developed a more sedentary life-style. At the same time, eating provided one of the few pleasurable experiences in otherwise dreadful circumstances. At the end of a year, I had gained 18 pounds. After the war, I traveled for a year, then settled into a comfortable teaching job, all the while eating more and exercising less. Within another year I was tipping the scales at 145 pounds, just like Sharon.

Looking back, Sharon undoubtedly could appreciate my embarrassment over being a 25-year-old fat physical education teacher who should have been setting quite a different example for her students, and she would understand why I chose an expedient solution, the so-called grapefruit diet. Supposedly, by combining a grapefruit with specific foods during each meal, my body would fight the calories in the other foods and help me peel off all those unwanted pounds. Sure, I lost some weight, but no matter how many hard-boiled eggs and grapefruits I gulped, I felt hungry all the time. Still, I had always been such a determined person, finishing anything I started, so I stuck it out. When I bet a friend I'd hit my weight goal by a certain date but found myself with 2 pounds and 12 hours to go, in desperation I donated a pint of blood to the blood bank, thinking that might do the trick.

I felt like a complete fool, having to resort to a stunt like that, and of course one pint of blood didn't do the trick, but that feeling put me back on the track. I began running moderately, only 1 mile a day. Gradually, I increased the distance to 2 miles a day, then 5, then 10, until I was competing in marathons. I followed Rule 2 for a while; then, when I hit my goal weight, I followed Rule 1 for a lifetime.

Do I *never* gain an ounce? Only a robot could claim such perfection, but when the demands of my business or a bicycle accident during a triathlon sideline me for a while and my weight begins to creep up again, I quickly regain my balance by eating somewhat less, then exercising again as soon as possible.

With my Slide Guide to keep a running count of calories and with my daily Personal Diet Calories Log and Exercise Calories Log, I can self-correct my weight within a week. So can Sharon. And so can you.

SHIFTING THE BALANCE

As you begin organizing your own personal program, bear in mind that a pound of fat equals 3,500 calories. Therefore, *if you wish to drop a pound of fat, you must create a 3,500-calorie deficit.* Don't try to do it too quickly, though. Remember that moderation is the key. You don't want to starve yourself, and you don't want to hurt yourself. Almost anyone can achieve a 7,000-calorie deficit (2 pounds of fat) a week, once the 500 calorie plus per day exercise and the 500 calorie minus per day diet levels are reached.

How many pounds do you want to lose? Do your Diet Calories Log and Exercise Calories Log balance? Can you safely decrease your intake by 500 calories per day? Can you increase your job, exercise, or other calories by a total of 500 calories per day? Suppose you are a woman who weighs 155 pounds but would like to reach 135 pounds within 3 months. You need to lose 20 pounds of fat, which at 3,500 calories per pound equals 70,000 calories. If you decrease your intake by 500 calories per day and increase your daily output by 500 calories, you have shifted the balance by 1,000 net calories. Thus, you could reach your weight goal in 70 days, or less than 3 months.

Before most of us can make equilibrium (Rule 1) a habit, we must make some major changes (Rule 2) in the way we eat and exercise. To make the necessary changes quickly and effectively, I recommend that you break down the change process into its component parts.

We're all creatures of habit, and we tend to become quite attached to personal routines that revolve around working, playing, eating, and sleeping. Taken together, our habits and commitments form our life-styles, the special mix of activity that stamps our lives with uniqueness. Of course, our habits and life-styles change over time, but consciously shifting them in a short period of time takes a lot of motivation, commitment, and ongoing reward. No changes require more willpower than shifts in eating and exercise habits.

Since the Equilibrium Plan inevitably demands shifts in these hard-to-change areas, I have tried to make the task more manageable by breaking Rule 2–type changes into two basic components: internal changes, which include perception, behavior, and life-style shifts, and external changes, which include everything in our environment.

Let's look at the internal changes first, beginning with your perception of yourself. Do you pride yourself on being a hearty eater? Some people treat eating as a burdensome necessity while others take great delight in it. Whether you are a gourmet or a gourmand, you should also look at food in terms of what's in it. Learn to differentiate good foods from bad. Read labels, multiplying the grams of fat times 9 calories and dividing it by the total number of calories to determine if it falls in the safe 25-percent range.

Pick good food over bad food, attacking any bad food habits by eliminating them one at a time from your diet. A massive assault on them may be too extreme. Gradual substitutions usually work best. Replace coffee with herbal tea. Substitute ice milk for ice cream, popcorn for crackers, and water for sodas. Eat smaller amounts more frequently. Learn to say no, not only to yourself but to well-intentioned relatives, hosts and hostesses who thrust an extra helping of pie à la mode onto your plate.

Reorganize your food choices to keep them within the 60%–25%–15% rule, letting these percentages govern your selections at the grocery store. Look for restaurants with menus that adhere to the 60%–25%–15% rule, and ask the waiter to leave the special sauce off your boneless chicken. You can tailor your fast-food orders by eliminating bad food items, and even first-class chefs will welcome your requests for a customized dish.

Do you define yourself as athletic? Lethargic? Somewhere in between? Believe it or not, each of us came into the world with innate athletic talent. Some individuals develop and display more talent than others, but no one need sit on the sidelines while others work out or compete in sports. You know the old saying that inside every fat person lurks a skinny person struggling to get out. Well, inside every sluggard lurks a runner, a dancer, a biker, a hiker, a competitor. Perceive yourself as an exerciser. See in every daily activity a chance to burn off a few more calories, be it walking an extra mile or parking at the back of the supermarket lot and walking a block to the store.

Perform your workouts at a certain time every day. Morning runs or walks burn off just as many calories as evening ones, so pick a time that suits your particular style and schedule. Make appoint-

ments with friends to exercise outdoors or at clubs so the commitment will add fuel to your resolve. Add variety to your workouts
by adding different activities or varying your schedule whenever
boredom sets in. Always go that extra mile. Do you dread climbing
the office stairs? Turn them into a personal gym, walking up and
down them two or three times a day with a vengeance.

Build a little adventure into your exercise program. Try a
new sport, something you have always wanted to do, such as
rowing a scull, wind surfing, rock climbing, parachuting, or scuba
diving. Build team sports into your weekends. Take a fitness
vacation rather than a resting vacation. Use your vacation time
to swim in new waters, hike through a national park, bicycle
along scenic byways.

Many of us work such long hours we often hire others to do jobs
around the house that could burn off valuable calories. Mow your
own lawn, wash your own windows or car, paint your own house.
Redefine chores as opportunities for a productive workout.

Your health is more important than anything in your life, so
every time you accomplish a change in your intake and output
of calories, reward yourself. Give yourself not only intangible
rewards (the good feelings you get seeing a slimmer reflection in
the mirror or being able to run 6 miles effortlessly) but also
tangible rewards that reinforce your Equilibrium Plan (a new set
of workout clothes or a new pair of running shoes).

What about external changes? As you progress toward your
weight goal, you will feel better and like yourself more. Talk
about these feelings with friends and relatives. Be proud of yourself and let it show. Others will share your improved self-image,
and their congratulations and encouragement can help you follow Rule 1 for a lifetime. If most of your friends like to focus on
food and parties rather than balancing these activities with sports
and recreation, make some new acquaintances.

Since we obtain a good deal of our perceptions of self-worth
from how others see us, we must sometimes alter our relationships with others so that our friends and social groups can help
us reach our goals. Seek out people who share your desire for a
more balanced life-style. Swim, bike, jog, or take a long walk in
the woods with a friend. Develop a relationship with someone
who will encourage you to stick with the changes that will bring
your caloric intake and output into equilibrium. If you're not a
joiner, connect with a fitness buddy. If you are, join a workout

club or a swimming, biking, running, walking, dancing, or hiking club, surrounding yourself with people who seek greater fitness. Teams, from softball to bowling, can provide wonderful companionship and reinforcement. Fitness-conscious friends and social groups can bestow tangible and intangible rewards. Compliment those who have made progress toward their weight goals or, better yet, give them a piece of sports equipment or treat them to a picnic that includes a workout.

Do you live in an area that encourages workouts—near a river, a bike trail, a park, or a fitness club? If not, plan to visit such areas regularly. Do you keep indoor fitness equipment at home —stationary rowing machine, bicycle trainer, a weightlifting bench? If not, invest in some new exercise "toys." Remember, you want to create a stimulating environment of fitness.

That is especially true of your eating environment, particularly if you are a businessperson. The business luncheon or dinner consumes a lot of time and can wreak havoc with your equilibrium commitments. Try to avoid having meetings with meals. Not only do you then eat by the clock rather than by hunger, you end up eating more than usual. When you hear the familiar "let's get together for lunch," suggest a different meeting format, perhaps including a walk. Schedule formal meetings before 11:30 or after 2:00.

If you eat out a lot, tell the person taking your order exactly how you want your food prepared and how much you'd like to see on your plate. When I dined with Nathan Pritikin, author of *The Pritikin Promise* and founder of the Pritikin Longevity Centers, he told the waitress, "Please take the salt and pepper shaker off the table with the ashtray, and bring fruit salad supreme without the whipped cream and without the liqueur, baked potatoes without any fixings, and the chef salad without the olives, sour cream, ham, or eggs."

PATIENCE PLUS PERSEVERANCE EQUALS PROGRESSION TOWARD PERMANENCE

To maintain equilibrium for a lifetime, it might help to remember the four p's: patience plus perseverance equals progression toward permanence.

Don't expect overnight miracles. People who have successfully lost and kept off weight for a long period of time all agree that they did not become fit and slim overnight. You learn how to run a 10-kilometer race by first running 1 mile successfully. You learn to eat nutritious food by learning what's in one food item at a time. Only gradually can the mind and body accept shifts and make them permanent.

But take heart. The Equilibrium Plan shows you how to lose 2 pounds (7,000 calories) of fat per week. That means 28,000 calories a month! At the end of 1 week you can measure your gradual progress on the scale or in the mirror, and at the end of 1 month you can hold 8 pounds of flour in your hands and actually see how much fat you've shed.

I've struggled with patience and perseverance myself. When I entered my first triathlon competition in 1978, I knew little about the sport other than that I needed a bike and a swimsuit. Grabbing my 10-year-old bathing suit, dusting off my ten-speed clunker, and donning my Nikes, I embarked on the Davis Triathlon, one of the few that starts with a run. I led the entire way, but after 3 miles on the bike I heard a whoosh as the first lightweight racer passed me at nearly twice my pace. I lost over 50 places before I began the final swim stage. Without goggles, swim cap, or wet suit, I hit the 62-degree lake with my body temperature well over 100 degrees. The rescue boats picked me up before I reached the halfway point in the swim. Hypothermia. Not only didn't I finish the triathlon, I spent the next several hours shivering uncontrollably. If I had had patience, I would have trained in a pool, tested the lake waters in advance, bought the right equipment, and trained on my ten-speed. I would have finished the race; I might even have won. That thought has helped me persevere and keep on entering endurance contests.

Our generation has witnessed an extraordinary number of changes. As the information age sweeps us into the world of artificial intelligence and robotics, I must continually remind myself that the human body will never change as fast as the world around it, but, as it reproduces itself, that remarkable bit of biology will outlast any spaceship or spacesuit we can design. That thought, too, keeps me persevering toward lifetime fitness.

If obesity were as frightening as cancer, you would probably do anything to "cure" it. But being overweight takes years to work its damage, and it takes years of patient persistence to cure. Bring your determined perseverance to both sides of the fitness equation. Don't cut calories too fast, and don't start working out too vigorously. In the long run, all your small, slow, moderate steps will grow into the permanent large one: lifetime fitness.

In Vietnam I learned a lesson in perseverance from the Asians who persevered against the chemicals of Agent Orange and the deadly fire of Cobra jet helicopters and B-52s. Racing on the trails of the Western States 100-Mile Race, I recalled that lesson when I, too, wanted to quit. At mile 85, in the dark of the night, after 22 long hours of running in the cold and the heat, a voice in my head said, Sally, it's OK to quit. You can always come back next year. It really doesn't matter, does it? You really didn't train enough anyway. What do you say when those voices ask you those kinds of questions? Do you sometimes hear your inner self say, It's OK to miss a workout, you can train tomorrow, or, It's OK to eat that fried doughnut or that hot fudge sundae. One piece won't hurt. When I hear those voices, I reach down deep inside myself to reserves of strength that can conquer those urgings, and I maintain control.

As you patiently persevere, changes will accumulate gradually, but over time clear progress will become apparent. Every long journey begins with a single step and involves innumerable additional steps before you reach your goal. The journey to your ideal weight progresses calorie by calorie, and along the way you pass many important milestones. By establishing small, achievable goals, you can constantly measure your progress. If you measure small quantities of diet and exercise calories (50 calories in a salad dressing or 50 calories burned off washing windows), you will gain great satisfaction as the small quantities gradually add up to large ones (50 portions of salad dressing grow to 2,500 calories, a full day's worth of eating, and 50 window washings equal a marathon run).

I like to race triathlons because they allow me to enjoy multiple finish lines. The end of the swim stage leads me to the starting line of the bike stage, and as I pass under the bike finish line, I reach the starting line for the run. At the end of the run, I cross the final finish line. The Equilibrium Plan works the same way, providing multiple finish lines and a grand finale reward: lifetime fitness.

Remarking on New England weather, Mark Twain once said, "If you don't like it now, just wait a few minutes." Throughout our lives we experience changes as we mature, change jobs, raise families, and fall victim to the tendency toward creeping obesity. Some changes you can control; others you can't. But the Equilibrium Plan puts you in charge of weight changes for a lifetime. If you follow Rule 2 to reach your weight goal and then follow Rule 1, you'll extend that progression to permanent fitness.

The notion of permanence hit me full force when my mother died from breast cancer after fighting for her life for 4 years after chemotherapy and a mastectomy. During that time my own doctor found two lumps in my breast. I had them removed immediately. My doctor advised me to stop drinking coffee because of the suspected link between coffee and cancer. It took me a year of quitting and starting again and quitting and starting again to finally kick the habit. So, even if you suffer some backsliding, as I do, as you engage in your own personal Equilibrium Plan, remember that you still hold the controls in your own hands, and one or two or three setbacks do not condemn you to ultimate failure. Permanent changes take time, and some of the most satisfying successes are born out of failure.

To conclude this midbook pep talk, let me dispose of some myths that may still be lingering in your mind about fatness, dieting, and exercising. These myths are age-old and still popular. If you can replace them with hard facts, you will start your own Equilibrium Plan on the right foot.

DIET MYTH BUSTERS

Myth: Obesity is inherited—I was born to be fat.
Fact: Although you may inherit tendencies, you do not inherit obesity itself. Genetically, you have inherited the shape of your body. Anyone can change his or her amount of muscle or fat. People, inadvertently or not, *choose* to be fat.

Myth: Obesity is caused by food allergies.
Fact: There is no proof that cytotoxic testing, a scientific technique for assessing food allergies, even helps determine which foods cause your allergies. The FDA and the American Academy of Allergy and Immunology call these tests gimmicks.

Myth: Fat people eat more than thin people.

Fact: Many thin people eat more than fat people because they exercise more and often choose foods not just according to the number of calories but according to the nature of those calories. To get slim and stay healthy, you can actually eat more volume if you exercise more.

Myth: Fat people lack willpower.

Fact: Lack of self-discipline in and of itself does not increase your body size or your body's percentage of fat. Fundamentally, obesity comes not from overeating but from not balancing the two sides of the fitness equation.

Myth: Emotional problems make you fat.

Fact: People don't get fat from emotional problems, but they do get emotional problems from constantly struggling and failing to lose weight. Emotions don't contain calories but they do cause a use of calories that can create fat.

Myth: Fat people are lazy.

Fact: Fat people are sedentary, not lazy. Fat people may lack the stamina required to move about like their more athletic, slim counterparts.

Myth: Ignore hunger.

Fact: Pay attention to hunger—like pain, it is sending your brain an important signal. It's not a matter of giving in to hunger or distracting your mind from it, hoping it will disappear. It won't. Feed your hunger with the quality foods and nutrients your body requests.

Myth: Hunger soon after eating indicates a psychological addiction to food.

Fact: No, but your body is flashing an urgent message—interpret it. It's not unusual, especially if you ate a high concentration of refined sugars, to feel hungry quickly (remember the sugar blues). Evaluate what you just ate. Did you feed yourself bad foods that often spark recurring hunger attacks?

Myth: To lose weight, you must severely cut back on calories.

Fact: No. Severely cutting back calories slows down your metabolism (a fact we will discuss in the next chapter). If you merely cut back on your calories, you will lower your basal metabolic rate almost the same amount. You won't lose fat.

Myth: A calorie is a calorie.

Fact: In terms of energy, all calories are equal. However, the *quality* of food makes as much of a difference as the *quantity* of calories. Each calorie differs from another in terms of its interaction with other calories. For example, a calorie of fat doesn't affect you the same way as a calorie of refined sugar, which signals the body to release insulin.

Myth: Effective dieting requires precise calorie counting.

Fact: Equilibrium does not depend on precision. To reach a new equilibrium point, you must offset intake with output. Until you appreciate the caloric and nutritional benefits and liabilities of good and bad foods, you can keep track of calories with the Equilibrium Plan Slide Guide.

Myth: You must be on a diet to lose weight.

Fact: Popular diets don't work in the long run. Calorie-reducing diets only restrict the number of calories you eat and decrease your physical energy level. Rather than diet, you should adopt a plan that includes healthy exercise and eating habits.

Myth: You must never eat "forbidden" foods.

Fact: If you eat and exercise properly, of course you can eat forbidden foods. You must be aware that some foods don't provide the same benefits as others, but if you are willing to pay the price, you can cheat.

Final Fat accumulates when the body does not burn excess
Fact: calories. In Chapter Six we'll find out just how to go about burning them.

EXERCISE MYTH BUSTERS

Myth: Fat people are heavier than skinny people.
Fact: That depends on what you mean by heavy. Fat people float in water, while fit people, carrying a high percentage of muscle, sink. Fat people's bodies are not as dense as skinny people's.

Myth: Fat turns to muscle when metabolized.
Fact: Wrong. Fat turns into something the muscles can burn: free fatty acids (F.F.A.). Fat cells can't turn to muscle because they only store fat and glycerol molecules. Muscle cells burn free fatty acids.

Myth: Fat-looking people are obese because they don't exercise.
Fact: You can't judge fat or skinny by appearance alone. You must also measure percentages of fat weight and muscle weight. Big people can look fat but carry a big, fit body, while skinny people can look thin and carry a weak, high-fat-percentage one.

Myth: If I run 10 miles at 6 minutes per mile, I'll burn more calories than if I run 10 miles at 8 minutes per mile.
Fact: Not true. You burn the same number of calories if you run the same distance.

Myth: Exercising will redistribute my weight.
Fact: Fat cells cannot be moved, only filled up or depleted. Muscle fibers can increase in size and become larger or smaller, but they certainly cannot move to different parts of the body.

Myth: By exercising, I can melt fat from my stomach.
Fact: Never. The melting point of fat is 300+ degrees and your body temperature is 98° F. You don't melt fat as you would in a saucepan—you burn it off by expending calories. There is also no such thing as spot reduction. You burn off fat according to how it was laid down: Last down, first off.

Myth: Exercise must hurt to count—no pain, no gain.

Fact: Wrong. To burn off fat, you must exercise at a moderate pace. Intense exercise burns off carbohydrates. Moderate exercise burns off fat. If you feel pain, you've made no gain.

Myth: More is better.

Fact: But too much is worse. You can overdo exercise, suffering injuries, burnout, and fatigue. You need to allow time for your body to rest and rebuild muscle tissue. Moderation is the key.

Myth: Quick weight loss is possible.

Fact: Possible, but not lasting. To lose fat permanently, you must combine an eating program with an exercise program, the only combination that provides lasting weight loss.

Myth: Exercise takes too much time.

Fact: A 1-hour daily workout takes less time than eating. The average American woman spends 4 hours per day buying, preparing, consuming, and cleaning up from eating. So it's worth spending an extra hour consciously exercising.

Myth: If I exercise, I want to eat more.

Fact: Intense exercise does create hunger drives because it lowers your blood sugar level, which triggers your hypothalamus, which, in turn, causes hunger pangs. Moderate exercise burns fats, lowers your fat levels, stabilizes your blood sugar levels, and acts as an appetite suppressant.

Myth: I was born fat and can't change.

Fact: Not on your life. When you were born, you had a certain number of fat cells. And today you can only fill them or empty them. The Equilibrium Plan will help empty them.

Myth: Exercise bores me to death.

Fact: Exercise comes in many exciting forms. Exercise should be play and play should be fun. The Exercise-Side Starter Program will help you develop invigorating and enjoyable exercises.

CHAPTER 5

THE DIET-SIDE STARTER PROGRAM

TEN RULES OF GOOD EATING

Before we look at some sample menus that will help you control the diet side of the fitness equation, we need to review some ground rules. By building a few basic rules of good eating into your diet, you will be able to benefit from healthful menus without starving or boring yourself with dull, unappetizing meals.

1. Eat less fat. Fat enters our diet two ways: in the processed foods we eat or in the food we prepare at home. I recommend that you restrict your fat intake to 42–75 grams per day. The ideal diet should adhere to the 60%–25%–15% rule, so you should cut your fat calories to 25 percent of your total calories. The following are acceptable levels of fat:

- For a 1,500-calorie diet, no more than 42 grams (1.5 ounces) of fat per day.
- For an 1,800-calorie diet, no more than 50 grams (1.8 ounces) of fat per day.

- For a 2,100-calorie diet, no more than 58 grams (2.1 ounces) of fat per day.
- For a 2,400-calorie diet, no more than 67 grams (2.4 ounces) of fat per day.
- For a 2,700-calorie diet, no more than 75 grams (2.7 ounces) of fat per day.
  Note: these levels are *not* appropriate for children under the age of two, who need milk fat and other fats in their diets for growth.

Successfully cutting back fat involves paying attention to what foods we buy and how we prepare them, as we saw in Chapter 2. Obviously, we can achieve the most significant fat cutbacks if we pay more attention to the meat in our diets.

Trimming fat off meat, avoiding cooking with animal fats, eating more lean chicken and fish instead of other meats, and ordering leaner cuts in restaurants can go a long way toward reducing your overall fat intake.

The same holds true for baked goods. Replace your cookie jar with a container of presliced fruit or vegetables, and when your birthday rolls around, celebrate with a fruit pie rather than a triple-layer double chocolate cake with fudge frosting.

Cheese deserves a special note because over the past 75 years Americans have increased their use of cheese from 5 to 26 pounds per person per year. Apparently we love cheese, putting it on our hamburgers and on our pasta, taking it on picnics, and devouring it at parties.

But 73 percent of the calories in most cheeses comes from fat. Most cheeses contain a lot of added sodium, and hard cheeses contain cholesterol. On the other hand, cheese is a great source of protein, calcium, and several vitamins. How can we keep it in our diets despite its fat and sodium content? First, treat cheese with respect by using it in limited amounts:

- Sprinkle instead of slice.
- Buy part-skim (lower-fat) cheeses when you can.
- Remember, just 1½ ounces (or ¼ cup of grated cheese) equals an 8-ounce glass of milk (1 milk-group serving.)

2. Avoid simple sugars. On the average, each of us consumes 128 pounds of sugar each year, or 600 blank calories per day. Surprised? That's because sugar comes to us in hidden form, often packed as the leading ingredient in processed foods and canned goods, the main ingredients of which aren't essentially sweet. White sugar contains 45 calories per tablespoon, brown sugar 52, and honey 61. The additional vitamins and minerals you obtain from honey or molasses (except blackstrap molasses, which offers a good deal of iron and calcium) do not offset their bad-food liabilities.

Smart dieters avoid adding sugar to their food, and they constantly search out and eliminate hidden sugar. Food manufacturers can cleverly disguise sugar by assigning it other names. Beware if you see any of the following names on a label, especially in first or second place (not counting water): sucrose, dextrose, fructose, maltose, glucose, any type of sweetener, such as corn syrup, brown sugar, raw sugar, or honey. Fruits canned in syrup may list corn syrup as the second ingredient; fruit punch may show sugar and corn syrup as the first ingredients; fruit yogurt will often reveal sugar as the second ingredient; most granola bars display sugar as the second ingredient; packaged pudding lists it as the first ingredient; and frozen fruit and juice bars frequently list it as the second ingredient.

Be especially careful with breakfast cereals. Some cereals mention sugar in the name of the cereal itself, while others disguise it under different names. The genuine "breakfasts of champions" contain high fiber, complex carbohydrates, and low sugar. Look for labels that offer those ingredients. Shredded wheat, puffed rice or wheat, plain corn flakes, and other plain rice and wheat products weigh in at acceptable levels. While many so-called natural breakfast cereals have come onto the market, you should be aware that the raisins and dried fruits in them also contain natural sugar.

3. Reduce salt intake. As with fat and sugar, salt or sodium often hides itself in our food. Indeed, while the American adult takes in an average of 5,000 milligrams (mg) of sodium each day, only a fourth of this amount occurs naturally in food; the rest comes from processed or canned foods and from seasonings, relishes, and table salt. The RDA for sodium is approximately 2,000–3,000 mg per day, depending on your level of activity. Only long-distance athletes can exceed that intake.

The 20th century has so conditioned us to prefer high salt (high sodium) diets that when we first reduce our salt intake, we often notice a difference in the flavor of our foods: lettuce becomes sweeter, meat duller. After a time, though, you will retrain your taste buds to appreciate the more natural flavors of your food.

As with sugar, many food manufacturers disguise salt with other names. Look for these sodium words: monosodium glutamate (MSG), sodium saccharin, sodium benzoate, garlic salt, onion salt, sea salt, brine (a mixture of salt and water), and nitrates. Manufacturers use sodium nitrites and nitrates to preserve foods, especially such meats as ham, bacon, sausage, hot dogs, and bologna.

Most fast-food franchises, and indeed many first-class restaurants, lace their foods with heavy doses of salt. Further, most frozen and canned foods, snacks, and spreads, such as ketchup, rely heavily on salt. By all means reduce your intake of such salty foods, but when you do eat them, never add extra salt to what's already there. Some people salt their food before they even taste it. Don't.

The following tips will help you reduce your salt intake at home:

- Buy water-packed tuna or salmon, rinsing it under cold water to remove some of the salt. Look for low-sodium choices in your store.
- Eat little or no processed luncheon meats, ham, sausages, salami, and pâtés (they also contain a lot of fat).
- Make your own soup stocks or buy low-sodium broth.
- Since some *medications* contain a lot of sodium, including such antacids as baking soda, opt for the low-salt types.
- Try low-sodium cheeses, which also contain less fat.

Further, you can replace salty seasonings with more healthful substitutes. Instead of salt and MSG, use herbs and spices, lemon juice, vinegar, tomatoes, garlic, or onions. Replace garlic salt with garlic powder, fresh garlic, or bottled garlic. Replace onion salt with onion powder, dried minced onions, or fresh onion. When using soy and teriyaki sauce, choose low-sodium types or dilute with wine or juice. To tenderize meat, rather than sprinkling on a prepared meat tenderizer, cook foods in a liquid (such as wine or chicken broth) and pound tough meats with a cubed hammer or buy them preground.

4. Eliminate or reduce caffeine. Kick the caffeine habit. If you consume more than 250 mg of caffeine per day, you are ingesting an addictive poison that can lead to nervousness and restless sleep. Though we most commonly associate caffeine with coffee, we can find it in lots of unexpected places, such as medications and soft-drink products. Chocolate, coffee, tea, cocoa, many soft drinks, diet pills, no-sleep pills, some aspirins, and other medications are loaded with caffeine.

The body needs water, and you may be surprised that a conscious daily consumption of 8–12 glasses of cold water will reduce your need for other types of drinks. However, if you have grown accustomed to drinking caffeinated fluids, gradually eliminate them.

- Instead of drinking coffee or caffeinated tea all day long at work, restrict yourself to one cup in the morning and one in the afternoon. Visit the water cooler when you crave something to drink.
- Rather than regular coffee, drink brewed decaffeinated or half caffeinated and half decaffeinated.
- Drink herbal or decaffeinated teas.
- Drink fewer regular and diet sodas in general, but select decaffeinated colas whenever possible.

5. Reduce or avoid alcohol. Athletes frequently ask me whether I recommend beer as a good pre- or post-event fluid. I always answer, "Of course not!" Alcohol provides no nutrients, and a 12-ounce can of beer contains the same amount of alcohol as, and 50 percent more calories than, a 1½-ounce shot of whiskey. As a diuretic, beer dehydrates you. After a workout, which has already left you in a dehydrated state, beer hardly makes sense. In Chapter 2 we saw all the health and calorie costs of alcohol, but if, despite these good reasons for not drinking alcohol, you still want to drink, try to limit the amount by following some of these suggestions:

- Try rotating between alcoholic and nonalcoholic drinks, such as mineral water with a slice of lime or lemon.
- Order "virgin" drinks (virgin piña coladas or daiquiris or Virgin Marys) or ask bartenders and hosts to make yours light.
- Order light beers or wine spritzers (wine and club soda) instead of hard liquor.
- Beware of wine coolers. While companies market them almost like soft drinks and even produce some in plastic liter bottles, coolers actually contain about the same amount of alcohol per serving as straight wine but with twice the number of calories.

6. Eat more complex carbohydrates. The healthful diet includes plenty of fresh vegetables, cereals, fruits, and grains. To increase your intake of complex carbohydrates, you can:

Eat more fruits:
- Store plenty of your favorite juices in the refrigerator for a breakfast drink or a snack.
- Choose a piece of fruit for an afternoon snack.
- Keep fresh frozen or canned fruits in the house as a late-night snack or dessert.
- Choose dried fruits, such as raisins or dates, as a substitute for sugar-rich treats.
- Eat lower-fat desserts, such as peach cobbler, fig bars, or apple crisp, rather than pies, cakes, and cookies.

Eat more vegetables:
- Refrigerate precut raw vegetables—carrots, cucumber, and celery—in water for salads and snacks.
- Mix cooked vegetables into your entrée, adding vegetables to any pasta dish, mixing some with your burritos or tostada, and adding them liberally to pizza.
- Add more types of vegetables, such as zucchini, red peppers, beans, peas, and squash, to your salads.

Eat more grains:
- Add grains to every meal. Eat pancakes, hot or cold cereal, toast, or bagels for breakfast, and include rice, bread, potato, or pasta in your lunch and dinner.
- Add grains as snacks. Munch on a bagel, English muffin, bowl of cereal, raisin bread, or cornbread for between-meal snacks.

7. Eat more fiber. The average American consumes only about 10–15 grams of fiber per day but should be taking in three times that amount, or 30–45 grams. Our low fiber levels generally indicate that we eat too much fat. High-fat dairy products and meats lack fiber. Fruits, vegetables, and whole-grain foods contain a lot of fiber, and you can obtain even more from unprocessed whole-grain foods, such as brown rice, oats, cornmeal, and wheat flour. Bran is loaded with fiber and can make very appetizing cereals, breads, and muffins.

Fiber makes up the connective tissue in plants, and while the human body cannot digest it, it nevertheless enhances the digestive process. You need plenty of fiber because:

- Fiber fills up your stomach, making you feel fuller after a meal.
- Fiber occurs naturally in healthful foods.
- Fiber may help tie up and remove cancer-causing substances.
- Fiber attaches to water, adding bulk in your intestinal tract, which helps move food waste out of your body, thus reducing constipation.

8. Drink 8–20 glasses of fluid each day. Why don't we drink more water? Probably because no commercial enterprise promotes this pure and inexpensive fluid. But water is the healthiest fluid you can drink. The fancier versions with minerals or carbon dioxide bubbles might be more entertaining, but ordinary water works just as well and costs less. You should drink at least 8 glasses per day, but if you work out a lot or naturally perspire more than others, you should probably drink up to 20 glasses of water per day. On hot days, you'll need to drink more than on cooler days.

The exercising dieter should follow this water-drinking timetable:

WATER CONSUMPTION AND EXERCISE

Time	Amount
2 hours before event	2.5 cups
15 minutes before event	2 cups
15 minute intervals during a hard workout	0.5–1 cup
After event	Replace weight loss with fluids

Caffeinated, alcoholic, and sweetened drinks not only play havoc with your system but actually dehydrate you as well, so next to water, I recommend natural fruit drinks, because they provide energy, nutrients, and refreshment. If you want to reduce the calorie content of fruit drinks, try diluting them with 50 percent water. One of my favorite drinks is water with half a squeezed lemon on ice.

Such fluids as broth and some soups give you too much salt. Punch and artificially sweetened fruit drinks provide loads of calories and few nutrients. Most important, though, avoid low-calorie or sugar-free soda. "Sugar-free" soft drinks foster psychological dependence on sugar, whether the drinks themselves contain calories or not, because they nurture your desire for sweets and sweet drinks.

The following tips will keep you sipping good fluids all day:

- Always place a filled water glass next to you as you work.
- Keep plenty of fruit juice, cold water, herbal ice tea, or lemonade in your refrigerator.
- In your car, carry a thermos jug filled with a cold drink.
- When you exercise, take a full bike water bottle with you.
- If you're going to the tennis courts or playing field, take along a large jug of water and drink some on your breaks. Drink *before* you feel thirsty.
- Eat foods with a high water content: watermelon, oranges, cucumbers, and low-fat ice milk.
- Put lots of ice in calorie-full drinks, since ice dilutes the calorie concentration.

- Drink vegetable juices, such as tomato, which contain fewer calories than most fruit juices.

Always be aware that the calories in drinks add to your total daily intake. Good clean water, with its zero calories, should head your list of preferred drinks, while colas should sit at the bottom. Also, given the choice of eating an apple or drinking the equivalent calories in apple juice, always select the apple because the unprocessed fruit offers fiber.

9. Eat a variety of good foods. Your body requires over 50 different nutrients to stay healthy, but no single food contains all of the essentials. Therefore, you must select foods from all the food groups, making a variety of choices within each one. By eating a variety of foods, you will ensure that you supply your body with all of the necessary nutrients it needs to run smoothly.

THE SIX MODERN FOOD GROUPS: A DAILY GUIDE

I. Meat, fish, and eggs, which supply essential amino acids, B vitamins, iron, and minerals. No more than 2 servings each day
   1 serving = 2 ounces meat, or
              2 egg whites
   Choose: Poultry without skin, fish and shellfish, lean red meat, tuna or salmon packed in water
- Lean meats include: veal leg, chops, cutlets; baby beef, beef chuck, flank steak, round steak; lamb shoulder, chops, leg; pork leg (whole rump center shank)
- When using more than one egg, try removing one or two of the yolks (i.e., with a two-egg omelette, use two egg whites and one yolk). Eat no more than three yolks per week.

II. Dairy Foods, which provide calcium, B vitamin, vitamins A and D, and additional protein: 2 servings each day
   1 serving = 1 cup milk, or
              1½ ounces cheese, or
              1⅓ cups cottage cheese, or
              ⅓ cup ricotta cheese, or
              1 cup yogurt

Choose: Low-fat or nonfat milk products or buttermilk; evaporated skim milk instead of cream; lower-fat cheeses (ricotta, pot, farmer, mozzarella) but check the label since it should list part-skim or skim milk

III. *Grains, Breads, and Cereal Foods,* which produce carbohydrate, iron, fiber, and B vitamins: 4 servings each day
1 serving = 1 slice bread, or
       ¾ cup dry cereal, or
       ½ cup cooked cereal, or
       ½ cup cooked rice or pasta
Choose: Whole-wheat, rye, oatmeal, or pumpernickel breads; bagels, tortillas (nonfried), pita bread; pasta (especially whole-wheat types); low-sugar, low-fat, and low-salt hot and cold cereals
- Avoid croissants, doughnuts, coffee cakes, snack crackers, etc.

IV. *Fruit Foods:* at least 2–10 servings each day
1 serving = about ¾ cup oranges, grapefruit, cantaloupe, mango, papaya, strawberries, apples, peaches, berries, grapes, bananas
Choose: Fresh or unsweetened frozen and canned fruits

V. *Vegetable Foods,* which produce carbohydrate energy and supply fiber, Vitamin A and other vitamins, and minerals: at least 2–4 servings each day
1 serving = ¾ cup cooked or 1 cup raw, spinach, romaine and red leaf lettuce, cauliflower, kale, collard greens, corn, watercress, chard, eggplant, endive, broccoli, potatoes, asparagus, carrots, squash
- Avoid vegetables packaged with butter or cheese sauces.
- Don't add butter or margarine to cooked vegetables.
- Season vegetables with herbs, spices, or juices, or add your vegetables to your main entree.
Choose: Fresh or frozen vegetables with little or no salt or sugar.

VI. *Convenience Foods, Fluids, and Other:* Potpourri
- Convenience foods: Limit the servings, not to exceed 1 per day.

- Fluids: Unlimited amounts of pure water (8–20 glasses) plus other nutrient-dense fluids, like tomato juice, nonfat milk, and fruit juices in water.
- Other (sauces, gravies, sweeteners): As few as possible and in small portion sizes.
  Choose: Products with low salt, sugar, and fat.

10. Balance your intake with your output. Combined diet and exercise will help ensure long-term weight control. The right food balance will include 60% complex carbohydrates, 25% fat, and 15% protein, and the right calorie balance will depend on your Equilibrium Plan Slide Guide calculations.

- When you do eat more calories than you should on a given day, offset that intake with extra output. If you indulge in an extra candy bar, also indulge in an extra walk around the block.
- If you eat a large meal, eat two smaller meals that same day —anticipate your day's meals.
- Try writing down what time of day and why you ate—look for bad-food daily routines.
- Substitute an urge to eat with an exercise bout, like a 5-minute walk in the fresh air.
- Delay your appetite by telling yourself you'll eat after you finish a project, not in the middle when your appetite urges you to.
- If you snack, eat fresh fruit first and drink fluids.

Now you're ready to design a starter diet that will put you in charge of one side of the fitness equation.

THE EQUILIBRIUM PLAN STARTER MENUS

Together with Elaine Moquette, a registered dietitian with a master's degree in public health, I have designed 14 breakfasts, 14 lunches, and 14 dinners, each of which obeys the 60%–25%–15% Rule, and each of which has been chosen for its virtues of balance and variety. You can, of course, select among them to suit your preference.

BREAKFAST—Basic Foods   (1)

Oatmeal, 1 cup cooked
Raisins, ¼ cup
Low-fat milk, ½ cup
Sliced apple, about 1 whole
Orange juice, 8 ounces

Calories: 521
Percent Calories From

Carbohydrate: 80%   Fat: 10%   Protein: 10%

BREAKFAST—Basic Foods   (2)

Bran Chex cereal, 2 cups
Low-fat milk, 12 ounces
Raspberries, frozen, unsweetened, ½ cup
Low-fat cottage cheese, ½ cup

Calories: 613
Percent Calories From

Carbohydrate: 62%   Fat: 16%   Protein: 22%

BREAKFAST—Basic Foods   (3)

Raisin bagel, 1 toasted, 55 grams (1.9 ounces)
Neufchâtel cheese, 1 ounce
Blueberries, frozen, unsweetened, ½ cup
Low-fat cottage cheese, ½ cup
Orange juice, 8 ounces

Calories: 494
Percent Calories From

Carbohydrate: 57%   Fat: 21%   Protein: 22%

BREAKFAST—Basic Foods   (4)

Whole-wheat English muffin, 1, 58 grams (2 ounces) with 1
   tablespoon preserves
Fruit salad, 1 cup
Low-fat milk, 12 ounces

Calories: 504
Percent Calories From

Carbohydrate: 70%   Fat: 15%   Protein: 15%

BREAKFAST—Basic Foods   (5)

Banana nut bread, 1 slice, 50 grams (1.8 ounces)
Wheat 'n Raisin Chex cereal, 1 cup, with ½ cup low-fat milk
Melon, 1 cup

Calories: 463
Percent Calories From

Carbohydrate: 68%   Fat: 20%   Protein: 12%

BREAKFAST—Basic Foods   (6)

Cantaloupe or other melon, 1½ cups
Whole-wheat toast:
   1 slice, 28 grams (1 ounce), with 1 teaspoon butter sprinkled with
   cinnamon, or
   2 slices, spread with 1 tablespoon of preserves
Low-fat milk, 8 ounces

Calories: 524
Percent Calories From

Carbohydrate: 65%   Fat: 20%   Protein: 15%

BREAKFAST—Basic Foods   (7)

Raisin bread, 3 slices, 25 grams (.88 ounce) per slice, spread with 1½
  teaspoons butter, sprinkled with cinnamon
Applesauce, unsweetened, ½ cup
Nonfat milk, ½ cup

Calories: 421
Percent Calories From
Carbohydrate: 66%   Fat: 18%   Protein: 16%

BREAKFAST—Basic Foods   (8)

Shredded Wheat cereal, 1½ cups
Strawberries, fresh or frozen, ½ cup
Low-fat milk, ¾ cup

Calories: 347
Percent Calories From
Carbohydrate: 72%   Fat: 13%   Protein: 15%

BREAKFAST—Frozen Entrée   (9)

Pillsbury microwave buttermilk pancakes, 3
Syrup, 2 tablespoons
Honeydew melon, 1 cup
Low-fat milk, 12 ounces

Calories: 591
Percent Calories From
Carbohydrate: 72%   Fat: 16%   Protein: 12%

BREAKFAST—Restaurant   (10)

Waffle, 1, 9″ square
Strawberries, unsweetened, 1 cup
Orange juice, 1 cup

Calories: 369
Percent Calories From
Carbohydrate: 70%   Fat: 20%   Protein: 10%

BREAKFAST—Restaurant   (11)

Pancakes, 3, 4″ diameter each, with 2 tablespoons syrup
Egg, scrambled, 1
Orange juice, 1 cup

Calories: 475
Percent Calories From
Carbohydrate: 66%   Fat: 23%   Protein: 11%

BREAKFAST—Restaurant   (12)

Scrambled eggs, 2
Wheat toast, 3 slices, 28 grams each (1 ounce), with 2 tablespoons
    preserves
Tea
Fruit salad, ¾ cup

Calories: 603
Percent Calories From
Carbohydrate: 64%   Fat: 21%   Protein: 15%

BREAKFAST—Fast Food   (13)

Bagel, 58 grams (2 ounces), with 1 ounce cream cheese
Apple juice, 12 ounces

Calories: 398
Percent Calories From
Carbohydrate: 72%   Fat: 19%   Protein: 9%

BREAKFAST—Fast Food   (14)

Bran muffins, 2, 40 grams each (1.4 ounces)
Orange juice, 12 ounces

Calories: 362
Percent Calories From
Carbohydrate: 71%   Fat: 20%   Protein: 9%

LUNCH—Basic Foods   (1)

Pasta salmon salad:
  Crushed salmon, 3 ounces
  Pasta, 1 cup cooked
  Green beans, ¼ cup
  Peas, ¼ cup
  Low-calorie Italian dressing, 2 tablespoons
Peaches, 1 cup, packed in juice

Calories: 474
Percent Calories From

Carbohydrate: 58%   Fat: 18%   Protein: 24%

LUNCH—Basic Foods   (2)

Lentil soup, 1½ cups
Whole-wheat rolls, 2, 28 grams each (1 ounce)
Vegetables and dip:
  Carrots, ½ cup
  Broccoli, ½ cup
  Cauliflower, ½ cup
  Low-fat plain yogurt, ½ cup mixed with dried onion soup mix
Mineral water

Calories: 536
Percent Calories From

Carbohydrate: 66%   Fat: 12%   Protein: 22%

LUNCH—Basic Foods   (3)

Crab melt:
  Canned crab, 3 ounces with celery, onions, 1½ tablespoons low-fat
  yogurt
  Green pepper, ⅓ cup
  Grated low-fat mozzarella cheese, ¼ cup
  Large French roll, 1, 60 grams
Pear, 1
Zucchini sticks, raw, ½ cup

Calories: 484
Percent Calories From

Carbohydrate: 54%	Fat: 16%	Protein: 30%

LUNCH—Basic Foods   (4)

Tuna salad sandwich:
  Tuna, packed in water, 3 ounces
  Celery stalk, and green onions, ¼ cup
  Low-fat plain yogurt, ¼ cup
  Spinach leaves, ½ cup raw
  Whole-grain bread, 3 slices, 28 grams (1 ounce) each
Peaches, 1 cup fresh or packed in juice
Raw cauliflower and carrot sticks, about 1 cup total

Calories: 652
Percent Calories From

Carbohydrate: 59%	Fat: 13%	Protein: 28%

LUNCH—Basic Foods, Picnic   (5)

  Broiled skinless chicken, 2 breasts, about 3 ounces each
3-bean salad, 1 cup, with 2 tablespoons reduced-calorie Italian
  dressing
Whole-wheat rolls, 2, 23 grams each (1 ounce), with ½ ounce
  Neufchâtel cheese spiced with garlic and herbs
Apricots, 3

Calories: 739
Percent Calories From

Carbohydrate: 41%	Fat: 20%	Protein: 39%

LUNCH—Frozen Entrée   (6)

Weight Watchers' Baked Cheese Ravioli
Carrot, 1 raw, 7 ½" long
Pear, 1 medium

Calories: 413
Percent Calories From
Carbohydrate: 61%   Fat: 22%   Protein: 17%

LUNCH—Frozen Entrée   (7)

Lean Cuisine Zucchini Lasagna
French bread, 2 slices, 35 grams each (1.2 ounces), with 1 teaspoon
    butter, garlic
Pears, packed in juice, 1 cup

Calories: 361
Percent Calories From
Carbohydrate: 63%   Fat: 19%   Protein: 18%

LUNCH—Restaurant   (8)

Minestrone soup, 1½ cups
Whole-wheat rolls, 2, 28 grams (1 ounce) each
Salad:
    2 cups romaine lettuce
    Tomato, one medium, mushrooms, ½ cup, onion, ½ cup
    Low-calorie Italian dressing, 2 tablespoons

Calories: 408
Percent Calories From
Carbohydrate: 64%   Fat: 20%   Protein: 16%

LUNCH—Restaurant   (9)

Turkey breast sandwich:
  Whole-wheat bread, 2 large slices, 42 grams each (1½ ounces)
  Turkey, 2.5 ounces
  Tomato, lettuce, or sprouts, ½ cup
  Mustard, no mayonnaise
Pineapple juice, unsweetened, 8 ounces

Calories: 495
Percent Calories From
Carbohydrate: 64%   Fat: 10%   Protein: 26%

LUNCH—Restaurant   (10)

Chicken breast sandwich:
  Whole-grain bread, 2 slices, 23 grams each (.8 ounce)
  Chicken breast, 2 ounces sliced
  Mustard; lettuce, 2 cups; tomato, 1 medium
Vegetable soup, 1 cup
Roll, whole grain if available, 1, 28 grams (1 ounce)
Mineral or regular water with a slice of lemon

Calories: 439
Percent Calories From
Carbohydrate: 57%   Fat: 15%   Protein: 28%

LUNCH—Fast Food (McDonald's)   (11)

Hamburgers, small size, 2
Nonfat milk, 1 cup
  Bring from home:
1 banana
Raw zucchini and cucumber sticks, about 1 cup total

Calories: 720
Percent Calories From
Carbohydrate: 55%   Fat: 26%   Protein: 19%

LUNCH—Fast Food   (12)

Pasta and seafood salad, 2 cups
  Bring from home:
Salad: grated carrots, ½ cup, or your favorite vegetable
Pita bread, 1 whole

Calories: 685
Percent Calories From
Carbohydrate: 57.6%   Fat: 30%   Protein: 12.4%

LUNCH—Fast Food   (13)

Vegetarian pizza, 2 slices, 12″ pizza with green pepper, mushroom,
  and onions
Orange juice, 12 ounces

Calories: 631
Percent Calories From
Carbohydrate: 57%   Fat: 26%   Protein: 17%

LUNCH—Fast Food   (14)

Wendy's chicken breast sandwich, no mayonnaise
Green salad:
  Broccoli, ½ cup
  Garbanzo beans, ¼ cup
  Romaine lettuce, ¾ cup
  Reduced-calorie Italian dressing, 2 tablespoons
Unfiltered apple juice, 12 ounces

Calories: 593
Percent Calories From
Carbohydrate: 57%   Fat: 22.5%   Protein: 20.5%

DINNER—Basic Foods   (1)

Chicken breast, without skin, 1
  Broiled with:
    Pineapple, ¼
    Teriyaki sauce, 1 teaspoon
Broccoli, 1 cup
Snow peas, ½ cup
Brown rice, 1 cup cooked

Calories: 440
Percent Calories From
Carbohydrate: 60%   Fat: 10%   Protein: 30%

DINNER—Basic Foods   (2)

Vegetable fettucini:
  Noodles, 1 cup cooked
  Cauliflower, ½ cup
  Broccoli, ½ cup
Sauce:
  Butter, ½ tablespoon
  Low-fat milk, ⅓ cup
  Parmesan cheese, 1 tablespoon
Baked apples with cinnamon, 1 cup

Calories: 409
Percent Calories From
Carbohydrate: 64%   Fat: 22%   Protein: 14%

DINNER—Basic Foods   (3)

Fish (ocean perch), 3 ounces cooked weight, baked with lemon and garlic
Noodles, 1 cup, with 1 teaspoon butter
Parmesan cheese, ⅛ cup
Asparagus tips, ½ cup
Mandarin orange wedges, ⅓ cup

Calories: 403
Percent Calories From
Carbohydrate: 51%   Fat: 19%   Protein: 30%

DINNER—Basic Foods   (4)

Broiled fish, 3 ounces, with salsa and cilantro
Cornbread, 1 piece, 40 grams, with 1 teaspoon butter or margarine
Brown rice, 1 cup cooked
Green beans, ¾ cup

Calories: 497
Percent Calories From

Carbohydrate: 60%   Fat: 19%   Protein: 21%

DINNER—Basic Foods   (5)

Tofu/vegetable stir fry:
    3 ounces tofu
    ½ cup bok choy
    ½ cup broccoli
Sauce: 1 teaspoon sesame seed oil
    ⅓ cup white wine
    garlic
    1 teaspoon low sodium soy sauce
    Serve over: chow mein noodles
Grapes, 1 cup

Calories: 461
Percent Calories From

Carbohydrate: 63%   Fat: 21%   Protein: 16%

DINNER—Basic Foods   (6)

Fish Dijon:
Fish (ocean perch), 3 ounces cooked weight, baked with onion,
    green pepper, chicken broth, and Dijon mustard
Brown rice, 1 cup cooked, sprinkled with ¼ cup grated cheese
Asparagus, 1 cup

Calories: 634
Percent Calories From

Carbohydrate: 57%   Fat: 21%   Protein: 22%

DINNER—Basic Foods   (7)

Manicotti, 2 shells, total cooked weight, 87.1 gm (3.1 ounces)
    Stuffed with ⅓ cup low-fat ricotta cheese, ⅓ cup frozen spinach
    topped with ½ cup tomato sauce, 1 tablespoon Parmesan cheese
Steamed zucchini, 1 cup

Calories: 396
Percent Calories From

Carbohydrate: 60%   Fat: 20%   Protein: 20%

DINNER—Frozen Entrée   (8)

Tyson chicken à l' orange, with fruited rice pilaf
    (boneless chicken breast with mandarin oranges)
Asparagus, 1 cup
Nonfat milk, 1 cup

Calories: 415
Percent Calories From

Carbohydrate: 46%   Fat: 19%   Protein: 35%

DINNER—Frozen Entrée   (9)

Lasagna florentine, 1 serving
Nonfat milk, 1 cup
Lettuce (2 cups) and tomato (1 medium) salad, with low-calorie
    French dressing
Whole-wheat bread, 1 slice, 23 grams (.8 ounce)
Applesauce, 1 cup, unsweetened

Calories: 621
Percent Calories From

Carbohydrate: 65.6%   Fat: 12.4%   Protein: 22%

DINNER—Frozen Entrée (10)

2 Budget Gourmet entrées, Oriental Beef (beef with vegetables over rice)
Cottage cheese, ½ cup, with ½ cup pineapple

Calories: 697
Percent Calories From

Carbohydrate: 53%   Fat: 18%   Protein: 29%

DINNER—Restaurant (11)

Spaghetti:
    Pasta, 1 cup
    Tomato sauce with mushrooms, ½ cup
Salad:
    Romaine lettuce, ½ cup
    Cucumbers, ¼ cup
    Tomato, 1
    Reduced-calorie Italian dressing, 1½ tablespoons
Bread, 2 slices, 30 grams each (1.1 ounces), with 1 teaspoon butter

Calories: 532
Percent Calories From

Carbohydrate: 67%   Fat: 21%   Protein: 12%

DINNER—Fast Food (Taco Bell) (12)

2 tostadas
    Bring from home:
Blueberry nonfat yogurt, Weight Watchers', 8 ounces

Calories: 508
Percent Calories From

Carbohydrate: 60%   Fat: 20%   Protein: 20%

DINNER—Fast Food (Roy Rogers)   (13)

Roast beef sandwich, 1
Potato with broccoli, 1, without cheese sauce
Bring from home:
Low-fat plain yogurt, ¼ cup
Grated cheese, ⅛ cup

Calories: 507
Percent Calories From

Carbohydrate: 48%   Fat: 25%   Protein: 27%

DINNER—Fast Food (Arby's)   (14)

Roasted chicken breast, 1 piece
Plain baked potato, 1 medium
Bring from home:
Broccoli, ¾ cup
Low-fat yogurt, ⅓ cup
Pineapple chunks, juice-packed, 1 cup

Calories: 622
Percent Calories From

Carbohydrate: 53%   Fat: 13%   Protein: 34%

CHAPTER 6

THE EXERCISE-SIDE STARTER PROGRAM

FAIDO AND DO YOUR BEST

In July 1985, I finished second in the Ironman-Japan Triathlon (a 2.4-mile swim, 112-mile bike, and a 26.2-mile marathon) with a personal record time of 10 hours 55 minutes. During the race, I had an experience I'll never forget.

Along the grueling course, our hosts had placed hundreds of banners in Japanese, which I assumed were sponsors' advertising. Then 4½ hours into the race I saw the banner printed in English: "Do Your Best." As I read it, I thought, That captures the true meaning of sports and competition.

Dismounting from my bike and lacing on my Nikes for the marathon, I continued to think about that slogan. It motivated me to race harder. I really *did* want to do my best. Throughout the race the rain poured on the crowds lining the course, all of whom patiently applauded for endless hours. They kept yelling at us *"Faido! Faido! Faido!"* When I first heard *"Faido,"* I pictured my two dogs at home, a Weimaraner and an English

126

pointer. Or did *"Faido"* mean second place, my standing in the race?

When I crossed a moat and passed through the walls of a 15th-century Japanese castle to the finish line in just under 11 hours, I saw a giant outdoor movie screen flash my picture. I can still see myself 30 feet tall. I was happy, wet, and tired, but I couldn't rest until I found out about that "Do Your Best" banner and that word *"Faido."*

An English-speaking Japanese triathlete explained that the young people in Japan have adopted the slogan "Do Your Best" as their motto, even printing it on their clothes, schoolbooks, and stationery just as our teenagers might stick a popular rock hero on theirs. I found myself wishing Americans would adopt that slogan, because it could spur us to higher performances in everything we do. It could certainly enhance our efforts to achieve and maintain our ideal weight, especially when it comes to exercise. No one has perfect willpower, and no diet and exercise plan is perfect, either; but if you always try to do your best, you will not only feel good about yourself, you'll end up looking great, too.

I also asked my English-speaking Japanese friend about *"Faido."* She paused before she answered, " 'Faido' means 'to fight.' " I was startled! The race had taken place on the 40th anniversary of the atomic bombing of Hiroshima, an anniversary that had reminded me of my time in Vietnam and had consequently revived my strong feelings against war and fighting. While many people have compared sports to war, to me they have always meant the exact opposite. War involves defeating and killing your competition, while sport involves competing fairly and amicably so that everyone becomes a better human being.

The Japanese triathlete noticed my displeasure and seemed concerned. "To the Japanese," she said, "the word 'to fight' in this context means to fight back against the negative that is within you, the bad thoughts that can lead to your self-defeat."

I understood. *"Faido"* had been telling us to fight against any negative inner voices that might have been telling us that we didn't have to do our best. It urged us to fight when we were weakening from fatigue, to fight against the impulse to quit and try again another time.

I thought *"Faido"* should also become an English expression.

For the Equilibrium Plan to work, each of us must fight against the temptation to be careless with our bodies and put off until tomorrow what we should do today. With *"Faido"* we can defeat all those internal obstacles that prevent us from doing our best today and every day.

GETTING READY

Although we discussed diet first, you know that the Equilibrium Plan involves the simultaneous control over both sides of the fitness equation. Therefore, at the same time as you work to cut your daily intake by 500 calories, you will be striving to burn off 500 more calories every day with deliberate exercise routines. Remember the four *p*'s: *p*atience plus *p*erseverance equals *p*rogression toward *p*ermanence. You want to start exercising slowly, gradually stepping up your workout until a vigorous one becomes comfortable, easy, and enjoyable. How long it takes you to reach 500 calories depends on your current condition and your fitness history. Remember those internal changes I discussed in Chapter 4.

You will also want to keep variety in mind, varying the time of day you exercise as well as the length and intensity of your workouts. Later in this chapter I'll recommend ways to get the most from all that you do. Approach your calorie-burning program as you would an enticing adventure. As you grow stronger and fitter, you will extend your range, cycling in new areas, running through previously untraveled terrain, planning walks to include sites of historic or natural interest. Use your program to explore previously unused, unseen aspects of your world and yourself.

Also bear in mind the external changes discussed in Chapter 4. I strongly recommend what athletes often call the buddy system. Although I often run with my dogs, I also enjoy a human companion or competitor. Not just any buddy will do. Work out with someone with whom you can share mutual support, someone at your fitness level with whom you can progress. I enjoy a variety of training partners—one who likes running short, fast distances, one who loves biking hard, another who prefers early-morning runs, and another who swims like a fish. If you can't find a buddy at first, keep looking. Eventually you will find that a spouse, friend, relative, neighbor, or colleague wants to attain a new equilibrium weight, too. To enjoy your workouts even more, become a joiner. Exercise clubs can provide social reinforcement, and so can clubs for walking, swimming, cycling, running, skating, skiing, dancing, canoeing, wind surfing, or even bird watching. Training with someone else, even if you generally prefer solitude, keeps you training longer. Clubs also provide education. You will always find someone eager to answer your questions and teach you new techniques and routines. You'll make like-minded, fitness-conscious new friends, and develop a built-in support system. To find out about the clubs in your area, call your local sports shop, pick up a sports magazine, read the newspapers, ask someone you see working out, or call the recreation department or the YWCA/YMCA. Meanwhile, a radio headset can make up for the lack of "live entertainment" during your workouts.

As for time, *make* time. Divide your day into three 8-hour blocks: if you work 8 hours and sleep 8 hours, the other 8 hours is "your time." As you plan your time, create new ways to burn calories all day: Walk, don't ride; stand, don't sit; sit, don't lie down. If you organize your time as well as you do your 8 hours on the job, you will create plenty of time for exercise. Walk, skate, run, or cycle to work. On your lunch hour, hit the trails, or if you work in a big city, engage in the office workouts described later in this chapter.

You'll want to start today, not tomorrow, but before you do so, heed this warning: If you have a history of medical problems, if you smoke, or if you carry more fat than 50 percent of your body weight, you should get a medical checkup before you begin exercising. Also, if you experience chest pains or other abnormalities while working out, stop and get a checkup immediately. Even if you feel good but have remained more or less sedentary for a number of years, you could benefit from a clean bill of health from a sports physician (sports physicians are trained to diagnose and solve *any* medical problem, not only fitness-related ones).

You will also need to get organized. Organize your clothes. Do you need a new outfit or a pair of sports shoes? When the weather turns cold, purchase the right apparel so you can continue working out comfortably. Buy the right socks, tops, shorts, bras, gloves, hats, glasses, helmets, footwear, underwear, and outerwear so that you can both look and feel good. Organize your equipment: Purchase the racquets, skis, skates, bicycle, canoe, workout machine, or any of the other "toys" that make exercising more fun. Organize your facilities. Locate the nearest high school track, scenic bike routes, gyms, lakes, hiking trails, and swimming pools. Chart new routes for walking to work, and start looking at the world of sidewalks and stairs as more than convenient modes of transportation.

Finally, you should make warm-ups and cool-downs the first and the last step of each workout. Never start or end a workout abruptly, but always proceed gradually from less to more activity, and vice versa. Both your warm-up and cool-down should take 5–15 minutes. To warm up you can start the activity itself at a snail's pace. The same holds true for cool-downs, which alleviate muscle soreness and hasten the necessary recovery period. I recommend stretching before you work out, and the stretches later in this chapter will get you ready for (and help you relax after) almost any exercise activity.

THE F.I.T. FORMULA

Designing your individualized training program involves the careful combination of frequency, intensity, and timing.

I'll never forget sitting in my graduate exercise physiology class at Berkeley when one of my favorite professors, Dr. Jack Wilmore, explained the frequency concept with the chart that follows.

Maximum fitness requires exercising more than four times per week, but beyond that you achieve less striking results. To attain 85 percent of a sport's fitness benefits you need only train in that sport 4 days a week. Of course, competitive athletes train up to four times a day 6–7 days a week, but these athletes have driven themselves far beyond simple health concerns.

Beginners should *never* try to train 6–7 days per week. Like starvation diets, overzealous exercise can be disastrous. For those who have just started a program, such enthusiastic overachievement can lead to muscle and bone injuries, increased appetite, and destruction of equilibrium. Start with 2 or 3 days a week,

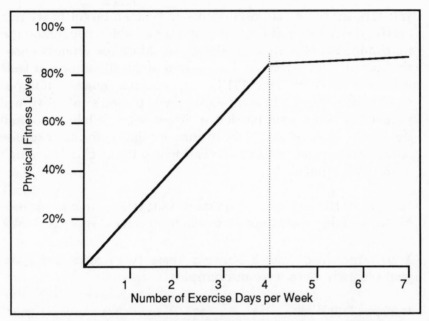

Frequency of One-Sport Exercise for Maximum Physical Fitness

gradually increasing to 4 days a week. With time and moderation, frequency will naturally increase and so will the calories you burn.

Dr. Wilmore also taught his students about sport-specific fitness. For example, if you train 4 days a week in tennis, you eventually become fit to play tennis, yet you will not necessarily become fit to play basketball. We can achieve two different kinds of fitness: cardiorespiratory fitness and muscular stretch/ endurance fitness. While most sports work the heart and lungs, each emphasizes a different group of muscles. That's why you should include more than one activity in your Exercise-Side Starter Program, strengthening more than one local muscle group.

You must also pay attention to intensity. Exercising too hard or not hard enough can retard your overall progress. You need to work out at an intensity level where you realize the greatest improvement, the level at which you work hard but still feel safe and comfortable. To determine the right intensity for you,

you can use pulse rate monitoring to reach a target heart rate (THR), the number of beats per minute at which you obtain the maximum benefits from working out. Most researchers agree that people who work out a minimum of 20–40 minutes at least 4 days a week at their THRs reap optimal benefits, but you can't reach that point overnight. Each person's intensity will reflect her or his own particular fitness level. While you could determine your exact THR by undergoing a formal exercise stress test in a laboratory, you can figure it out closely enough with this formula:

Maximum THR = 220 (your maximum heart rate) − your age × 80%
Minimum THR = 220 (your maximum heart rate) − your age × 65%

Your target heart rate is between these two figures. Using 38-year-old Jody Carper as an example:

Maximum THR = 220 − __38__ = __182__ × .80 = __146__ beats per minute
Minimum THR = 220 − __38__ = __182__ × .65 = __118__ beats per minute

Now, calculate your own THR:

Maximum THR = 220 − ____ = ____ × .80 = ____ beats per minute
Minimum THR = 220 − ____ = ____ × .65 = ____ beats per minute

Take your pulse by using a watch with a second hand. Count the number of heartbeats in 6 seconds, then add a zero to that number. If you count 13 beats in 6 seconds, your pulse rate is 130 beats per minute. You'll find the strongest pulse in your neck on either side of your voice box (the carotid artery next to the larynx). Until you can instinctively evaluate your THR in terms of how hard you're breathing, you should stop exercising every 5 minutes or so to take your pulse. If it falls below your target range, step up your activity. Your THR makes an ideal intensity gauge because it automatically adjusts for improvement. As you get generally fitter, so does your heart.

Finally, you want to stress timing, the T of the F.I.T. game plan, by considering the length of time you work out. Start with a shorter period of time, then gradually increase it. Step 1 of the Exercise-Side Starter Program begins at 50 calories, which you can obtain with 5 minutes of swimming, 9 minutes of cycling, or 10 minutes of moderate walking. Remember, start slowly and gradually increase the duration of your workout sessions. Within a week, your workouts will feel easier as your body adapts to slight equilibrium shifts. After a week, you should be able to increase your exercise time by at least 20–50 percent. You will be up to half an hour of exercise quite quickly.

You will experience the most dramatic changes during the first 6 months as your body gets stronger and your exercises seem easier and easier. Your idle speed will increase, your appetite will decrease, your desire for good foods will take hold, and your body shape and image will improve markedly toward your ideal. Eventually, you will stabilize at a new and lower equilibrium weight.

EQUILIBRIUM GAME PLAN

So far we have talked about what everyone should do before, during, and after engaging in exercise activities. Now you want to tailor a program to meet your own needs and preferences. Before you do so, consider how Mike Bell went about it. He weighs 170 pounds and likes to play badminton, which the Slide Guide tells him burns 225 calories per half hour for a man of his weight. To burn 500 calories, he would have to play for about an hour and a quarter. Given the principle of gradualness, I would advise Mike to start at 50 calories per workout if he's unaccustomed to exercise and at 100 per session if he's in reasonably good shape. In the case of badminton, an unfit Mike would play 7 minutes at his THR to hit the 50-calorie goal, while the fairly fit Mike would play for 13.3 minutes at his THR to reach the 100-calorie goal. But how do you know whether you're fit or not?

Fitness defies easy definition because, like "happy" or "depressed," it includes a full spectrum or continuum of states. On the bottom of the continuum lies the danger zone, which can lead to disease and debilitation; on the top lies a plane of ideal physical well-being and optimum good health.

However, exercise physiologists have established a battery of fitness tests, called the physical performance profile, that measures fitness levels rather precisely. These profiles include strength, flexibility, cardiorespiratory condition, muscular endurance, and body composition (percent fat/muscle and lean weight). You can obtain a comprehensive medical evaluation of your fitness. Many of the HMOs (health maintenance organizations) include this within their health insurance coverages. But let's assume you rate your own fitness components on the Five Levels of Fitness scale.

· If you have not routinely followed an exercise program during the past year, you should probably begin as an Ironperson of Step 1. Remain at that level until the level of activity feels comfortable. When the current level becomes easy, you can then move up to Step 2 and become a Steelperson. After a minimum of 2 weeks at that level, you may proceed to the next level, entering Bronze, after which you can progress slowly, but painlessly, to Silver and Gold. If you have been exercising regularly, you may start higher, possibly at Silver. Select any of the activities listed on the Equilibrium Plan Slide Guide or in the Appendix and enter it on your personal Equilibrium Game Plan.

FIVE LEVELS OF FITNESS

Level	Calories per Workout	Time (minutes)	Frequency (days)	Time on Plan
1. Iron	50	5–10	3–5	2–8 weeks
2. Steel	100	10–20	4–6	2–6 weeks
3. Bronze	200	20–30	5–6	2–4 weeks
4. Silver	350	30–45	6	2–4 weeks
5. Gold	500	45–60+	6–7	Lifetime

Let's watch Mike Bell use his Equilibrium Game Plan to lose 24 pounds in 12 weeks. Mike played sports in high school. In college he played seasonal intramural flag football, basketball, and softball. Graduating from college as a fit 5-foot 9-inch, 150-pounder, he began the career treadmill, which just didn't seem to allow time for working out. Married, with two children, he worked 50-hour weeks and spent the weekends playing with his kids and watching football on TV. His midriff had begun to bulge, and over the last two decades he had tried to fight creeping obesity with diet sprees that only fed his fat cells even more.

By the time he turned 40, he weighed 174 pounds. Since his

father had recently survived a heart attack, Mike knew that he also ran a high risk of heart disease, even though he didn't smoke. He wanted to get back into shape. Though he suspected a connection between his weight and his eating/exercise balance, he did not have a clear grasp of the problem until he went on the Equilibrium Plan. He allowed himself 3 months to get into shape. After all, what are 3 months compared to 20 years of slowly advancing obesity? And what are 3 months compared to the next 13 years, when he would enter a new century at age 54?

Defining his current self-image and projecting a fitter one with the Chart on page 15, he tackled the diet side of the equation with a 60%–25%–15% carbohydrate, protein, and fat diet that eventually reduced his daily calorie intake by 500 calories. Then he designed his own Equilibrium Game Plan, gradually building his output to 500 more calories per day. Ultimately, then, he created a daily deficit of 1,000 calories per day. Since his intake averaged 3,000 calories per day, he would have to cut this by 700 calories, then add 100 calories with exercise, 100 calories with job calories, and 100 calories in other activities to create his 1,000-calorie-per-day deficit, and shed 2 pounds of fat weight per week. If he worked up to 500 exercise calories a day, he would be able to eat more calories and still maintain a 1,000-calorie deficit. Watch as Mike progresses from Iron to Gold on the game plans shown on the following pages.

Mike alternated days and always took his rest day between exercise days. He could have worked out 4 days back to back, but he knew he needed to give his muscles time to rest and his body time to build more muscle tissue before working out again.

Mike also cycled and walked at his target heart rate, stopping every couple of minutes to check his pulse. Since he spent 5 minutes warming up and 5 minutes cooling down, his total workout time took 16–17 minutes, not much when you think about it. But those 50 calories a day really added up.

After one week, Mike found this exercise program so easy he moved on to the Steel level.

On the Steel level, Mike maintained the same warm-up and cool-down periods but added a day of exercise to his routine, and he dropped the cycling in favor of swimming. He also went from walking briskly to jogging mildly. At this point, Mike began notic-

EQUILIBRIUM GAME PLAN

NAME: _____Mike Bell_____   DATE: _____May 1, 1987_____

Body weight: Present: _____174_____   Goal: _____150_____

Activities: __Walking__
                   __Cycling__

F.I.T.: Frequency: __2__ days per week each activity

Intensity: __117 to 144__ heartbeats per minute (THR)

Timing: __5__ minutes warming up

__8__ minutes at THR for walking

__7__ minutes at THR for cycling

__5__ minutes cooling down

Weekly Workout Schedule

Level: Iron

Day	Activity	Calories per Half Hour	Number of Minutes	Calories Burned
Monday	Walking	198	8	53
Tuesday	REST			
Wednesday	Walking	198	8	53
Thursday	Cycling	231	7	54
Friday	REST			
Saturday	Cycling	231	7	54
Sunday	REST			

Total calories burned per week **214**

EQUILIBRIUM GAME PLAN

NAME: _____**Mike Bell**_____ DATE: _____**May 8, 1987**_____

Body weight: Present: _____**172**_____ Goal: _____**150**_____

Activities: **Jogging**
 Swimming

F.I.T.: Frequency: **5** days per week

Intensity: **117** to **144** heartbeats per minute (THR)

Timing: **5** minutes warming up

10–20 minutes at THR for each activity

5 minutes cooling down

Weekly Workout Schedule

Level: Steel

Day	Activity	Calories per Half Hour	Number of Minutes	Calories Burned
Monday	Jogging	315	10	105
Tuesday	REST			
Wednesday	Swimming	294	11	108
Thursday	REST			
Friday	Jogging	315	10	105
Saturday	Swimming	294	11	108
Sunday	Jogging	315	10	105

Total calories burned per week **531**

ing distinct changes in his body. He had lost an inch around his waistline and his pants fit better. Sure enough, after 2 weeks as a Steelperson, Mike had lost another 4 pounds, bringing his total to 6 pounds. Not only was he shedding fat weight, but his eating habits were giving him more strength, as he ate more carbohydrates to fuel his muscles. Though he couldn't see it happening, his mitochondria energy factories were increasing, thus allowing him to burn more fuel.

After 2 weeks at this level, Mike was ready to tackle Bronze. Again, he decided to test out new activities, this time high-energy aerobics and tennis.

Mike discovered that he loved the aerobics class, where a roomful of high-energy people shared the common goal of fitness. But tennis challenged Mike. He had learned to play in high school but had quit after college. Once he found a partner, though, the skill came back quickly. In tennis, as in his other sports, Mike always burned a few extra calories by bending over to pick up the ball rather than picking it up with his racquet or by walking fast after the point to get in position for the next serve.

After another 2 weeks, Mike had gained so much confidence that he decided to try some new activities: running, basketball, and riding on a stationary bike. Basketball would improve his eye-hand coordination, running would get him outdoors, and he could set up his stationary bike in front of the TV. Exercising was becoming a habit, but, more important, it was becoming fun. See how Mike planned his Silver level exercise program.

After seven weeks on the Equilibrium Plan, Mike had dropped 14 of the 24 pounds of fat he wanted to lose and had gained muscle, interesting new sports activities, and friendships with like-minded people. Finally, he could go for the Gold. Having spent two weeks at each prior level, for a total of eight weeks progressing toward Gold, Mike stuck with this program for four weeks. In 12 weeks he reached his ideal weight of 150 pounds. He bought new clothes to match his improved self-image and decided that he liked himself more, now that he was eating good foods/good calories and exercising regularly. Put together your own program tailored to your professional and family commitments and to your personal exercise choices. Mike's game plan only works for Mike. Yours will work for you.

EQUILIBRIUM GAME PLAN

NAME: _____**Mike Bell**_____   DATE: _____**May 22, 1987**_____

Body weight: Present: _____**168**_____   Goal: _____**150**_____

Activities: __**Aerobics (high)**__
__**Tennis (singles, recreation)**__

F.I.T.: Frequency: __**5**__ days per week

Intensity: __**117**__ to __**144**__ heartbeats per minute (THR)

Timing: __**5**__ minutes warming up

__**20–30**__ minutes at THR for each activity

__**5**__ minutes cooling down

Weekly Workout Schedule

Level: **Bronze**

Day	Activity	Calories per Half Hour	Number of Minutes	Calories Burned
Monday	Aerobics	366	15	183
Tuesday	REST			
Wednesday	Aerobics	366	15	183
Thursday	Tennis	231	15	115
Friday	Aerobics	366	15	183
Saturday	REST			
Sunday	Tennis	231	15	115

Total calories burned per week **779**

EQUILIBRIUM GAME PLAN

NAME: ___Mike Bell___   DATE: ___June 5, 1987___

Body weight: Present: ___162 pounds___   Goal: ___150 pounds___

Activities: ___Running (9 minutes per mile)___
___Basketball (full court game)___
___Cycling on stationary bike (15 mph)___

F.I.T.: Frequency: ___6___ days per week

Intensity: ___117___ to ___144___ heartbeats per minute (THR)

Timing: ___5___ minutes warming up

___30–45___ minutes at THR for each activity

___5___ minutes cooling down

Weekly Workout Schedule

Level: Silver

Day	Activity	Calories per Half Hour	Number of Minutes	Calories Burned
Monday	Basketball	420	25	360
Tuesday	Stationary cycling	366	29	353
Wednesday	REST			
Thursday	Running	447	25	373
Friday	Stationary cycling	366	29	353
Saturday	Basketball	420	25	360
Sunday	Running	447	25	373

Total calories burned per week 2,172

EQUILIBRIUM GAME PLAN

NAME: _____**Mike Bell**_____   DATE: _____**June 19, 1987**_____

Body weight: Present: __**160 pounds**__   Goal: __**150 pounds**__

Activities: __**Aerobics (high)**__
__**Cycling on regular bicycle (13 mph)**__

F.I.T.: Frequency: __**6–7**__ days per week

Intensity: __**117**__ to __**144**__ heartbeats per minute

Timing: __**5**__ minutes warming up

__**45–60**__ minutes at THR for each activity

__**5**__ minutes cooling down

Weekly Workout Schedule

Level: Gold

Day	Activity	Calories per Half Hour	Number of Minutes	Calories Burned
Monday	Aerobics	330	50	550
Tuesday	Cycling	330	50	550
Wednesday	Aerobics	330	50	550
Thursday	REST			
Friday	Cycling	330	50	550
Saturday	Aerobics	330	50	550
Sunday	Cycling	330	50	550

Total calories burned per week **3,300**

EQUILIBRIUM GAME PLAN

NAME: _____   DATE:_____

Body weight: Present: _____   Goal: _____

Activities: _____

_____

_____

_____

_____

F.I.T.: Frequency: _____ days per week

       Intensity: _____ to _____ heartbeats per minute (THR)

       Timing: _____ minutes warming up

                   _____ minutes at THR for each activity

                   _____

                   _____

                   _____

                   _____

                   _____ minutes cooling down

Weekly Workout Schedule

Level: _____

Day	Activity	Calories per Half Hour	Number of Minutes	Calories Burned
Monday	_____	_____	_____	_____
Tuesday	_____	_____	_____	_____
Wednesday	_____	_____	_____	_____
Thursday	_____	_____	_____	_____
Friday	_____	_____	_____	_____
Saturday	_____	_____	_____	_____
Sunday	_____	_____	_____	_____

Total calories burned per week .... _____

WARM-UPS

As we saw in Chapter 3, the total number of calories you burn each day includes more than exercise. While you can boost your total calorie burning most dramatically with exercise, you can also increase the number of calories you burn on the job or while engaged in other activities. The fourth category of calorie burning, your idle speed, will automatically increase as you shed fat and gain muscle. Let's see how we can squeeze out as many calories as possible from all that we do.

Your warm-up, lasting about 5–10 minutes before each workout, prepares your body for exercise by lubricating your joints, lengthening your muscles and tendons, and gearing up your cardiorespiratory system. For many sports, a mild form of the activity will get the job done. Runners can begin by stretching, then walking, then slowly jogging up to speed; swimmers can wade through the water, stretching, floating, and performing underwater calisthenics (these burn extra calories because of the water's resistance); and tennis players can touch their toes, twist at the hips, and bounce the ball against a wall before taking on an opponent. Such snail's pace warm-ups will help prevent soreness and injury.

One of the keys to milking extra calories out of all your workouts is getting in touch with every muscle in your body. By concentrating on different sets of muscles, you will find some to which you've paid little attention in the past. At first, you may feel a little soreness there, but that will quickly go away as you shape up that area. The following basic stretches concentrate on limbering up specific sets of muscles:

Calf stretch. Stand facing a wall, 3 feet away, feet 12 inches apart. Extend your arms straight out, shoulder-width apart, and lean forward until your hands touch the wall. Keep your legs and back straight, heels on the ground, and let your elbows bend as you lean forward until your face touches the wall. Hold for 5 seconds. Straighten your arms as if you were doing a push-up. Repeat five times. You should feel the stretch in the back of your lower legs.

Groin stretch. Sit on the floor with your knees bent out to the sides, the soles of your feet touching each other. Sit with your back straight and your hands around your feet. Simultaneously pull your feet in toward your body and force your knees out and downward toward the floor. Then lean forward, lowering your head toward your feet. Repeat three to five times.

Side stretch. Stand up straight with your feet 3 feet apart, arms against your sides. Looking straight ahead and without bending forward, bend slowly to one side, keeping your arms as close to your leg and side as possible. Reach as far down one leg as possible, then repeat the same, slow motion on the opposite leg. Repeat three to five times in each direction.

Leg up. Stand facing a waist-high platform. Lift your right leg in front of you, placing your heel on the platform. Bending at the hips, lean forward with your upper torso toward the raised leg. Hold for 15–30 seconds. Repeat with the left leg. You will feel your hamstrings, the muscles on the back of your legs, stretch. Repeat three to five times.

Leg back. Lie on your stomach with your head resting on the floor. Reach behind with your right hand and grasp your right toe, pulling it toward your buttocks. Hold for 15–30 seconds. Repeat on the left side. Feel the muscles on the front of your thigh, the quadriceps, stretch. Repeat three to five times.

Reaching prayer. Kneel on your hands and knees with your knees spread about 6 inches apart, directly under your hips. Keep your hands and knees in position as you lower your buttocks until they touch the heels. Reach forward and lower your chest to the floor and hold for 15 seconds. Repeat stretch five times. It stretches the muscles of your lower back and hips.

Head roll. As you look straight ahead, press your left ear toward your left shoulder and hold for five counts. Keep shoulders down and relaxed. Press your right ear toward your right shoulder and hold. Feel the stretch in your neck. Now, slowly, roll your head in a complete circle in one direction, then in the other direction. Repeat three to five times.

Shoulder stretch. Standing straight, bend your right arm behind your head, reaching down your back. Take your other hand and apply pressure to your right arm, holding for 5 seconds. Repeat to the left side. Repeat three to five times.

Trunk rotation. Stand upright with your hands behind your head, feet about 3 feet apart. Rotate your trunk as far to the left as possible and hold for 5 seconds. Then rotate as far to the right as possible and hold. Repeat five times. You should feel the muscles in your back, sides, and shoulder areas stretch.

Bar hang. Grab a bar overhead with your hands, facing forward, and lift your feet off the ground, bending at the knees. Hang for 60 seconds. Feel the muscles in your arms, shoulders, back, trunk, and hips stretch.

I also recommend five total-body warm-ups, each of which involves both the upper and lower body as well as the extremities. Besides warming up your entire body, they allow you to pump up your cardiorespiratory system without any equipment, such as weights or a swimming pool. In fact, you can do them in your street clothes or business attire, and not just before you work out. You can also use them as first-thing-in-the-morning calorie burners, before you shower and get dressed for the day.

60-second marches. Starting slowly, walk forward with a marchlike step, lifting your knees high and pointing your toes forward. Perform a similar arm motion. Synchronize your arms with your legs, swinging the opposite arm and leg with each step. As you proceed, stretch your arms higher and higher until your hands reach for the sky. Move forward ten steps, then make a 90-degree turn, take ten more, turn another 90 degrees, and repeat the procedure until you complete a square. Gradually increase the height of the knee lift and the arm swing by stepping up on your forefoot.

60-second forward leaps. Leaping forward 2 feet per stride, extend one arm and the opposite foot. After ten leaps, lengthen the stride by 12 inches, then take another ten strides. Keep lengthening your stride until you reach your maximum. Do it again, but now aim for height rather than distance.

60-second jogging jacks. Perform a jumping jack with your arms while walking, then jogging, in place with your feet. Start with your arms at your side, then bring them up with your elbows straight and clap your hands above your head. Drop your arms and repeat, increasing the intensity of your footwork.

60-second circle shuffle. To the beat of an inner drum or a stereo, dance or shuffle in place as you slowly roll each body extremity 360 degrees ten times. Start with head circles, then make shoulder circles, until you've moved each part of your body. When you move your hips, imagine using a hula hoop.

Circle shuffles also develop your coordination and balance.

60-second push-up toe raises. Start in a push-up position, then walk your feet forward, with your hands in place. Press up high on your toes, then lower your heels five times. Now, with your back straight, walk your hands back to the push-up position. If you can, do a push-up or two, then walk forward again with your feet.

If you engage in these and other warm-ups four to six times a day, say before breakfast, before lunch, before a workout, before dinner, or as a change of pace during an office-bound or meeting-filled day at work, you will not only burn a few extra calories, you will be keeping your body limber and loose for all your activities, not just your formal workouts.

Seize opportunities for warm-ups. Believe it or not, your bed can help you burn more calories. No, I'm not talking about sex, though that of course can be a wonderful way of burning off calories. I'm talking about stretching yourself awake in the morning. After a good night's sleep you probably stretch and yawn automatically when you wake up, but try turning that unconscious habit into a conscientious workout. As you lie there, visualize each set of muscles, then concentrate on lifting and extending them. Start with your toes, pointing them down, then up. Lift each leg 3 inches and hold for 30 seconds. Reach for the ceiling, do a few sit-ups, twist your torso and neck. When you finally get up, you will find your body prepared for another high-energy day.

MORE EXERCISE CALORIES

All warmed up and ready to exercise, you can begin burning a few extra calories during your workouts, too. It just takes a little creativity and alertness. To get you started on the road to milking extra calories from your workouts, let's look at some of the exercises listed on the Equilibrium Plan Slide Guide.

Billiards. Not one of your most strenuous sports, but you can practically double its benefit while you're waiting your turn by holding your cue stick vertically against the floor at arm's length and "walking" your hands down and up it. Placed across your shoulders, it can help you twist your torso. Few of your playing partners will mind if you do a few deep knee bends or toe touches between shots.

Golf. Another sedentary sport for those who ride golf carts, it can provide many opportunities for extra calorie burning. Use a club the same way you would the pool cue. Walk briskly down the fairway, and when you reach your ball, bend from the hips to touch it five times. Carry your own clubs, and even add a few pounds of weight to your golf bag. Do some stretching exercises while you're waiting your turn at the tee.

Walking. Carrying extra weight really works wonders here. Turn your child into an exercise machine by carrying him or her in a backpack rather than pushing him or her in a stroller. If you push your child, walk briskly. If you don't have children, load a backpack with books or invest in inexpensive wrist and ankle weights offered by a number of athletic equipment manufacturers. Look for hilly terrain (a 5-percent grade can literally double your calorie output), and hike off the beaten path. Fields and hillsides, dirt roads, sandy beaches, and grassy tracks will require more effort than the mundane asphalt. Perhaps you've seen race walkers competing in the Olympics and thought they looked silly. Without looking silly, you can double the speed of your walking to double its benefit, provided you still walk the same length of time.

Running. Of course, you can speed your walk to a run, and you can increase your calorie burning with hills, sandy beaches, and some added weight on your wrists and ankles. In some cities, competitive racing up the stairs of skyscrapers has become a fad. You may not want to run to the top of the Empire State Building, but even a three- or four-story stair run burns triple the calories of a flat surface run over the same distance.

Aerobic dancing. Stand in front of the class, where you'll feel more pressure to keep pushing than if you hide yourself in the back. Wear wrist or ankle weights, or hold a pair of 1- to 3-pound Heavyhands while whirling through your workouts. At home, play music with a faster beat. If you watch one of the morning wake-up shows, video-tape some programs so you can work out again later in the day. By the way, *any* kind of dancing, except the cheek-to-cheek kind, burns lots of calories. Schedule dancing after dining, and if you feel shy, a dance class can give you skill and confidence.

Tennis. Bend over to pick up the ball, run to your position, touch your toes or do deep knee bends between games, bounce on the balls of your feet before your opponent serves. Look at your racquet and your tennis ball as more than tools of the sport. Gripping each end of your racquet, raise your arms high, twist at the waist, touch your toes. Carry a tennis ball when you walk to work, squeezing it with either hand; store one in a desk drawer so you can toss or squeeze it while talking on the phone.

Bicycling. These wonderful machines allow you to create a whole world of extra calorie burning. If you ride a ten-speed bike, challenge yourself with higher gears on hills. Build hilly terrain into your touring, and carry extra weights on your wrists and ankles or in a backpack. Stand up to pedal. Remember those old single-speed balloon-tire bicycles? You can still buy inexpensive ones, or you can pick them up at flea markets and garage sales. Since such a bike takes a lot more work to ride because of its weight, use it occasionally to train for ten-speed riding. The new heavy-duty mountain bikes can get you off the well-traveled roads and into some beautiful, calorie-burning new scenery.

Stationary biking. Stationary bicycles have become quite popular, but many of them are collecting dust in basements because their owners quickly got bored with them. To combat boredom wear a personal stereo, read a book, or watch TV. Some video companies now offer interactive bicycle tours that will send you zooming through the Napa Valley wine country without leaving your living room, actually creating a visual bicycling experience that simulates the real thing. Strap weights to your ankles or wear a pair of heavy boots, and invite a friend to watch a rented movie while you share a satisfying workout.

You get the idea. Within every sort of exercise lurk opportunities to bend and stretch and twist or add weight. A good imagination will help you add 20 calories here and 50 calories there, and before long you can be gaining 5–25 percent more from every workout.

MORE JOB CALORIES

Your creative imagination can also put more calories into your job. Let's consider how the executive editor Jack Taylor might increase his daily output by as many as 500 calories.

Commuting by foot. Not only does Jack walk three-fourths of a mile to work each day, he always loads his briefcase with extra weight (books and the dress shoes he switches for his running shoes when he gets to the office). He's always in a rush in the morning, so he heads straight for the office, but at the end of the day he adds a half-mile loop to his walking commute home. Lately he's worn a pair of 2-pound ankle weights hidden beneath his slacks.

The coffee break workout. Since Jack works on the 17th floor, he hits the staircase for 15 minutes twice a day because he knows that even slow-paced stairwalking burns as much as three times the calories as strolling along a level surface. Usually he carries a heavy book in each hand or puts on his ankle weights.

The exercise meeting. His day fills up with long meetings around a conference table, but whenever Jack reviews the performance of one of his people or needs to have a long one-on-one conversation with a client or coworker, he tries to conduct it while walking. Of course, that was easier when he worked in the suburbs, but he's been pleasantly surprised by how many people enjoy a meeting more and solve problems more effortlessly outside the confines of a meeting room.

The prelunch workout. Jack has turned a lot of his colleagues on to an inexpensive piece of exercise equipment that tucks neatly under any desk and attacks that most troublesome portion of the anatomy, the stomach. It is a rubber wagon wheel with a steel axle that has handgrips on either side. To use it, you grip the axle in a kneeling position and push the wheel out as far as possible. When you pull it back, you lift yourself up with muscles in your abdomen. Just 10 to 50 a day help harden Jack's stomach, and it only takes him 5 minutes to do it. Luckily, his office has a door he can close. Otherwise he might feel self-conscious.

The calorie-burning business lunch. On the days when he hasn't scheduled a luncheon meeting, Jack walks to a grocery store and delicatessen to buy a good-food sandwich and a piece of fruit. Sometimes he eats in the park, chinning himself beforehand on the playground bars; sometimes he carries his lunch back to the office. When he has planned to meet someone for lunch, he makes reservations at a restaurant at least six blocks from the office. Occasionally he swims or plays racquetball during lunch hour, but he always treats lunch as a chance to burn off the calories he's eaten.

The afternoon workout break. In the middle of the afternoon, Jack closes his door, has his secretary hold his calls, and jumps in place for a few minutes. This invigorates him so much he has been thinking about buying one of those small, portable trampolines to keep at the office.

The "get it yourself" philosophy. Jack stopped expecting his secretary to bring him his coffee years ago, but he has also developed the habit of sharpening his own pencils, fetching his own files, emptying his own waste basket, and generally walking to get it himself.

Other businesspeople build similarly creative workouts into their normal workdays. Those who drive to work can consciously stretch arm, leg, and neck muscles when the car is stationary. Any stationary object, like a steering wheel, offers an opportunity for isometric exercises, involving gripping, tensing, and relaxing muscles. Take the handrails on staircases, for example. With your hand on the rail and one foot a step above the other, you can extend thigh and calf muscles. To stretch the back of your legs you can put one heel two steps above the other and bend forward until your chest touches your knees. When you talk on the telephone, work with a weight or stretch. If you type or input, add wrist weights and watch the caloric cost double.

Think of your steering wheel, your desk top, and your staircase as instant gymnasiums. Don't just sit at your desk all day, but periodically stand back a few paces with your hands gripping the edge and do several half push-ups.

Even people who enjoy outdoor jobs can fail to recognize all their opportunities for extra calorie burning. Added weights, a get-it-yourself philosophy, and an alertness for tasks and objects that can be turned into exercise opportunities abound for surveyors, gardeners, lifeguards, traffic cops, and meter readers. It all depends on making the unconscious conscious and keeping an eye open for chances to burn a few more calories with everything you do to earn a living.

MORE CALORIES FROM OTHER ACTIVITIES

We all engage in activities other than exercising or working, and they can offer some of the best opportunities for extra calorie burning. Every day we listen to music, watch TV, eat meals, drive our cars, putter around the house, pursue hobbies, and do all the other little daily things that make up our lives. In most cases, we can turn what could be sedentary activities into body movement. The more we move, of course, the more calories we burn.

Every movement has a caloric cost. It would be impossible for us to measure the calories burned by every single movement we make, but consider what a 130-pound woman normally burns doing what we classify as daily activity.

The figures represent averages, but you can improve them substantially by building more movement into them.

Card playing (45 calories burned per half hour). While reading your cards, lift your legs beneath the table, hold them there, then move your feet a few inches apart, then back together 20 times. While the dealer shuffles, place your hands on the sides of your chair, raise yourself from your seat, and hold yourself there for 30 seconds. Get up and move around between hands, touch your toes, do a few deep knee bends, and stretch your arms toward the ceiling and rotate your wrists. You could easily double your calorie burning.

Watching television (36 calories burned per half hour). Do you sit quietly while watching television? Try knitting or stretching. Stationary biking while viewing your favorite program could raise your calorie burning by as much as 20 times! You could do housework or perform any of the warm-ups mentioned earlier without hampering your enjoyment of television. If you watch a few hours a day, you could define that big chunk of time not only as mental relaxation or stimulation but also as a chance to burn up calories that would otherwise turn to fat.

Food shopping (111 calories burned per half hour). Park at the back of the parking lot. Rather than pushing your child in a stroller or shopping cart, carry him or her in a backpack. Heft large packages a few times, as you would dumbells, bend over for products on lower shelves, and stretch up to higher shelves. Carry your groceries to your car instead of pushing them in your cart, and perform a few warm-ups before getting into your car. That might look silly in the frozen-food aisle, but it would look quite normal in a parking lot, where joggers often warm up and stretch.

Vacuuming (81 calories burned per half hour). Your vacuum cleaner can become a piece of exercise equipment if you weave warm-up and stretching routines into your housekeeping chores. Bending, twisting, stretching, and reaching out vigorously into floor corners and high into ceiling corners can add calories to this humdrum task. Carry rather than roll your vacuum from room to room, and pause between rooms to do some toe touching, squatting, or rotating calisthenics.

Gardening (228 calories burned per half hour). All sorts of appliances and machines make our lawn work effortless, but sometimes we should prefer a little effort. Every other week use a push mower rather than power mower (if you have both) and trim the edges by hand, stooping over rather than using an electric trimmer. When you get down on your hands and knees to plant bulbs, use those motions to work out different muscle groups. Reach, lift, stoop, carry, push, and pull when you would normally use a stepladder, a wheelbarrow, or a rake. In the winter, forgo a snowblower for a good old-fashioned snow shovel.

Sex (135 calories burned per half hour). I'll leave this one to your imagination.

Regardless of how you spend your spare time, be it cooking or washing dishes or landscape painting or dog grooming, treat each activity as a chance to burn a few calories. Rely a little less on services you can hire and the appliances you can buy: Split your own wood, wallpaper your own den, rake your own leaves, pick your own apples, wash your own car. It may take a few more hours a week, but it could easily add years to your life.

COOL-DOWNS

You can use cool-downs (the same sorts or routines as you use to warm up) not just to ease yourself out of a workout but to help you to relax into a peaceful day's end. Review the warm-up section, then begin looking for ways to cool down not only at the end of the day but during the day as a welcome change of pace.

Cool-downs also offer a chance for greater creativity. After you climb into bed, stretch to relax yourself and ease the tensions of your busy day. You can also use your shower stall to unwind and burn a few calories to boot. Feel the water pass over your muscles as you place your hands against the walls of the shower stall. Bend from the lower back and press forward. Pull in your stomach for 30 seconds. Twist from the hips and rotate your spine. Raise your body on your toes and stretch a dozen times. Most cool-down stretches can be just as easily performed in a shower, when you get the added benefit of warm, relaxing water.

IDLE SPEED

As you increase your muscle percentage and decrease your fat percentage, you will grow and multiply more mitochondria, which leads to your being able to increase the calories you burn at your idle speed.

In the beginning, you won't see a dramatic change in your idle speed because it will be trying to maintain a constant equilibrium, but eventually with more muscle and less body fat composition it will move upward, provided you maintain your workout program. Remember, if you cut calorie intake without exercising, your idle speed will respond by slowing down.

Once you have raised your idle speed, you will be burning more calories while at rest, and those extra calories, added to your now higher levels of job, exercise, and other calories, will result in a snugly fitting spacesuit. As I promised at the beginning of this book, you will now be eating more volume (and more wisely) because you are exercising more (and more wisely).

Finally, we have prepared our spacesuits for the year 2000. However, before I wrap up our discussion of the Equilibrium Plan, I'd like to give you one more tool, perhaps the most important one so far, the Challenge Reward Chart, which will graphically track your progress toward lifetime fitness.

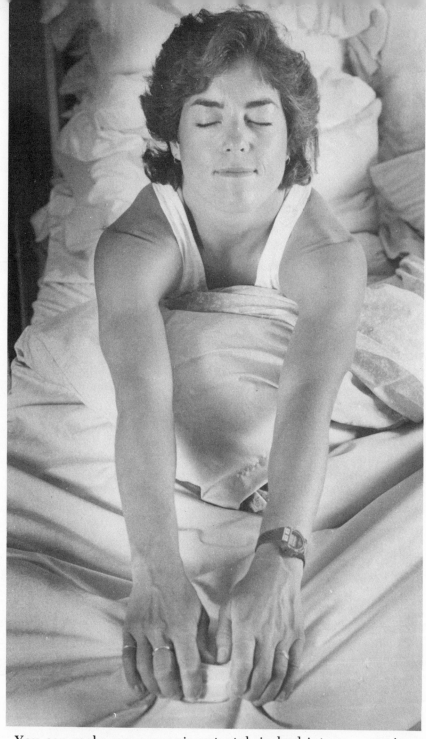

You can make your morning stretch in bed into an exercise before you even get up.

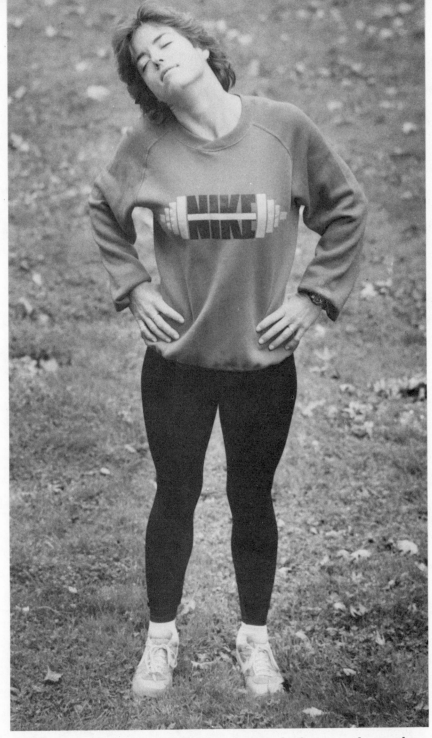

And you can do this warm-up exercise before you leave the house. Slowly roll your head, legs, and arms—one at a time— in circles. Repeat, rolling in the opposite direction.

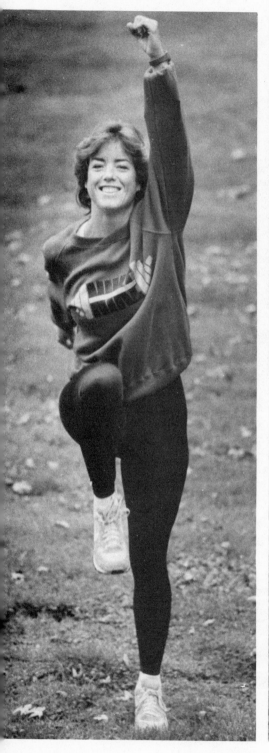
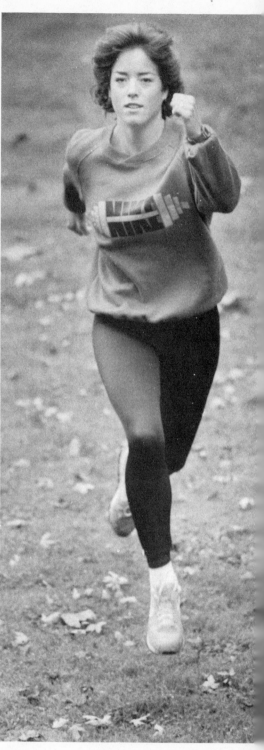

Three warm-up exercises. *March:* knees high, toes pointed. Stretch knees and arms higher with each step. *Foward leaps:* Stretch arms and feet further forward with each step. After 10 leaps, lengthen your stride. *Jogging jacks:* Jog in place, knees high, hands clapping over head.

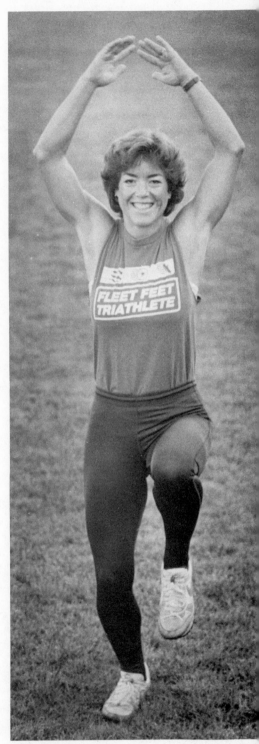

Push-up toe raises. Start in the push-up position, then walk forward, keeping your arms stationary. Press up high on your toes, then lower heels five times. Walk forward with your hands to the starting position.

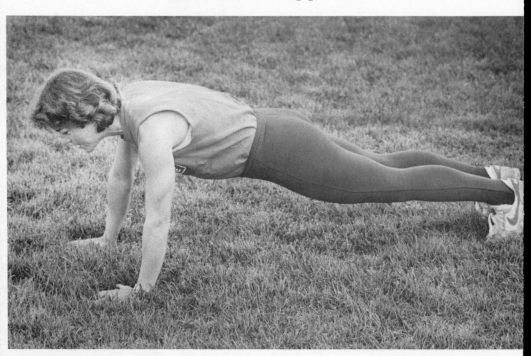

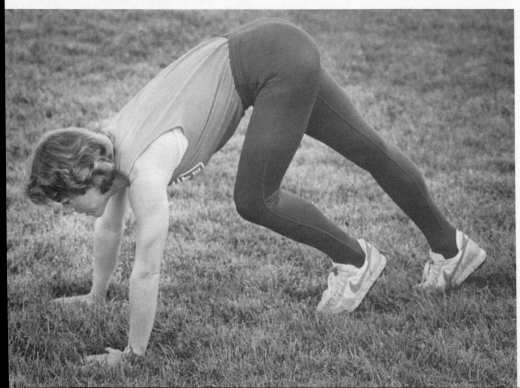

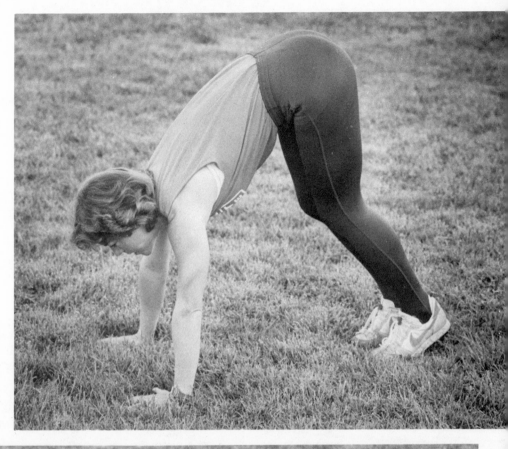

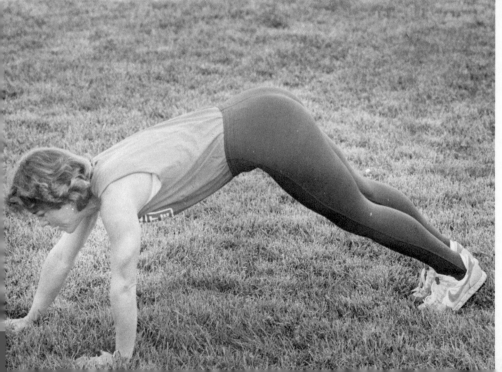

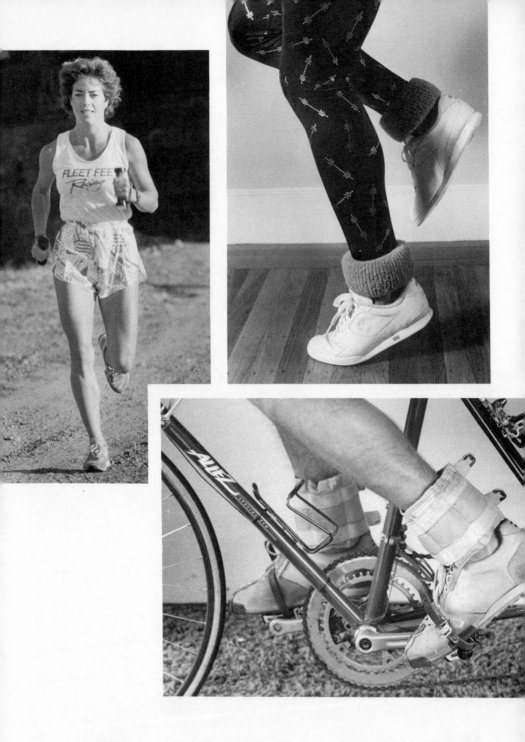

You can burn more calories if you add weights to your ankles and wrists when you run, during aerobic dancing, bicycling, at work, even washing the car.

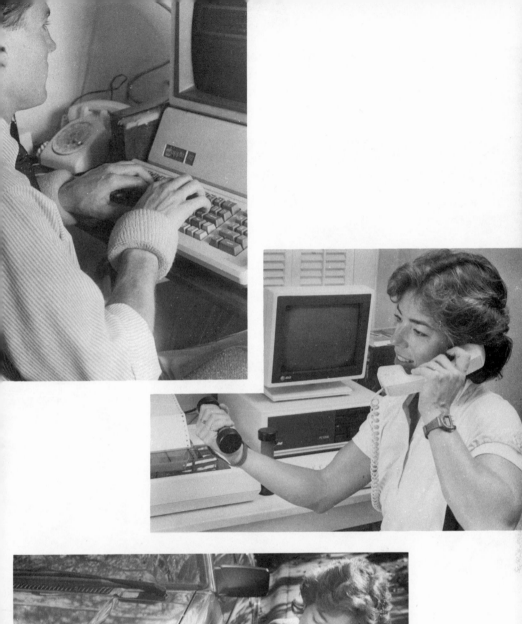
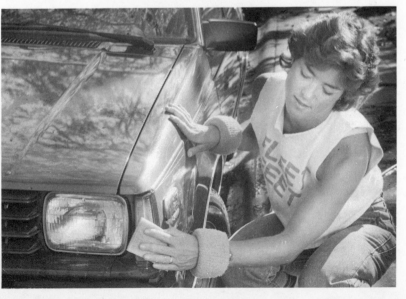

Look for ways to work off more calories in your favorite sport. Pick up the tennis ball, instead of scooping it up with your racket. Get off the saddle when you ride your bike, and take the hilly route home.

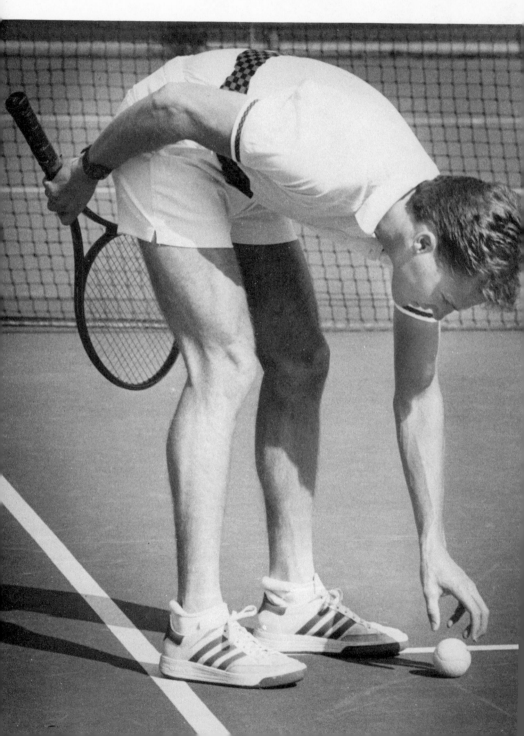

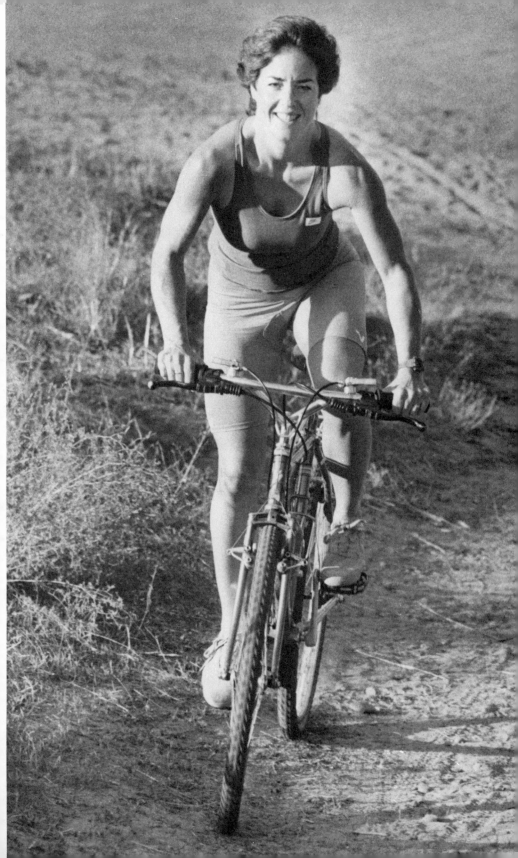

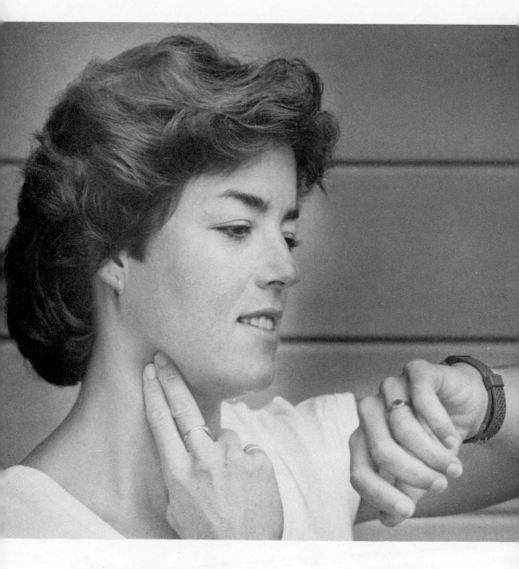

Take the carotid artery pulse for a good indication of how hard you are working out. Gently press under the angle of the jaw on one side of the midline of your neck. If you're working hard, you'll find the pulse easily. Count your beats for 6 seconds and multiply by 10.

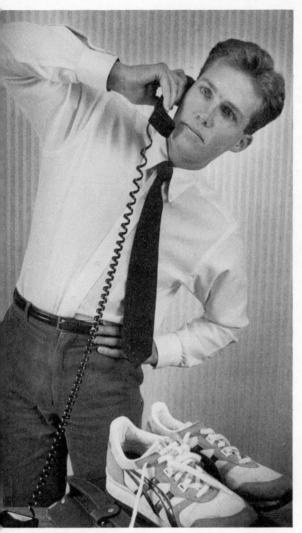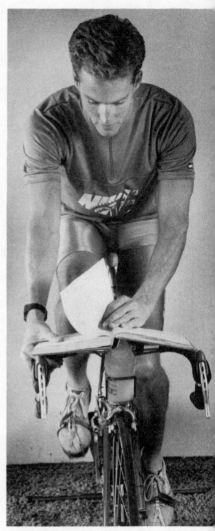

Stretch when you're on the phone. Exercise while you read or watch television.

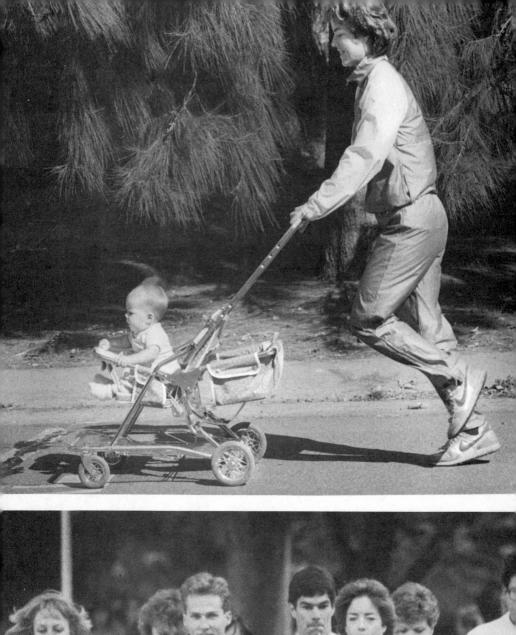
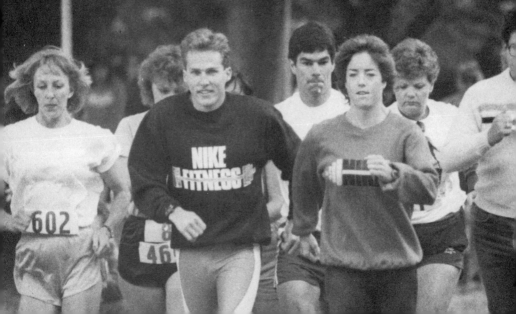

Taking your baby for a stroll burns calories. Taking your baby
for a run burns more.

Other people can be wonderful motivators.

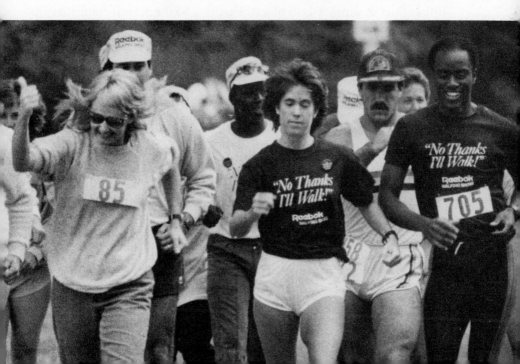

CHAPTER 7

THE
BIG
REWARD

RISKS AND REWARDS

When I competed in my first marathon in 1976, I crossed the finish line in almost last place. I paid a $20 entry fee and went home with a $5 T-shirt, a crippled knee joint, sore, cramped muscles, and bone-deep weariness. But I also took home a sense that I had accomplished something extremely important to my pride. I had finished, so to myself I had won.

Now a major marathon winner can earn a $50,000 prize, but whether I win or not, I still get a boost to my self-esteem every time I cross the finish line. The same holds true for my business. In the early days I worked long, hard hours just to break even, but no matter what the balance sheet showed at the end of the month, I felt a great sense of accomplishment from having struck out on my own. Now I open several new stores every year as my business generates more and more profits, but no amount of financial success can replace the exhilaration of knowing I have built something from scratch.

In sports and business, the rewards come in many different

forms. Some are symbolic: badges, pins, certificates, T-shirts, or plaques. Others are more tangible: money and the things money can buy. Still others are psychological: pride, self-esteem, public and private recognition. Similar awards will come your way as you begin winning the war on weight. In the early stages of your Equilibrium Plan, when your investment of time and effort seem highest, you will probably benefit most from the symbolic and tangible rewards, but when you break through to the point where you can actually see the results of your diet and exercise programs in the mirror and on the bathroom scale, you will gain even more reinforcement from the psychological rewards: feeling good about yourself, enjoying the way you look, and noticing the approval of friends and relatives.

Earlier we had talked about risk. Obviously, sports success and business success depend on competitors taking risks, but so does the success of your personal Equilibrium Plan. In our efforts to shed unwanted pounds, we can learn from the professional gamblers who control the one-armed bandits in Las Vegas. Sometimes I play the nickel slot machines. If you pump a paper cup full of nickels into the machine, you will occasionally hit a small jackpot, and these small, timely rewards will keep you popping in nickels and pulling the handle in the hope that the big jackpot will come with the very next tug. For your Equilibrium Plan to succeed, you need to develop a similar program of risks and rewards, using the small, intermediate milestones of a 2- to 10-pound weight loss or an effortless extra mile of running to keep you pushing toward that ultimate, and real, jackpot—a lifetime of fitness.

MILESTONES

To make a long-term commitment to anything as difficult as lifetime fitness, you need to pass a series of milestones on the path from the starting line to the finishing tape. These milestones should:

- Come early in your program
- Occur frequently
- Provide visual stimulation

- Offer symbolic reinforcement
- Bestow material gratification
- Accumulate toward the big reward

The Equilibrium Plan Challenge Reward Chart fulfills all of these requirements. It provides a daily and weekly record of your progress toward your ideal weight. It starts on Day One of your Equilibrium Plan; it allows for frequent reinforcement; it establishes a visual record; it rewards you symbolically; it gives you a concrete picture of your progress; and it builds toward the ultimate reward of lifetime fitness.

Let's see how Jack Taylor completed his Equilibrium Plan Challenge Reward Chart. Since a single chart encompasses only 14 days, Jack needed to fill out six charts for the 12 weeks it took him to go from 170 to 155 pounds at the recommended 2 pounds per week.

Notice the continual downward direction of Jack's weight,

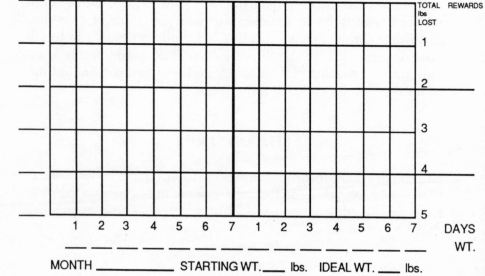

Challenge Reward Chart

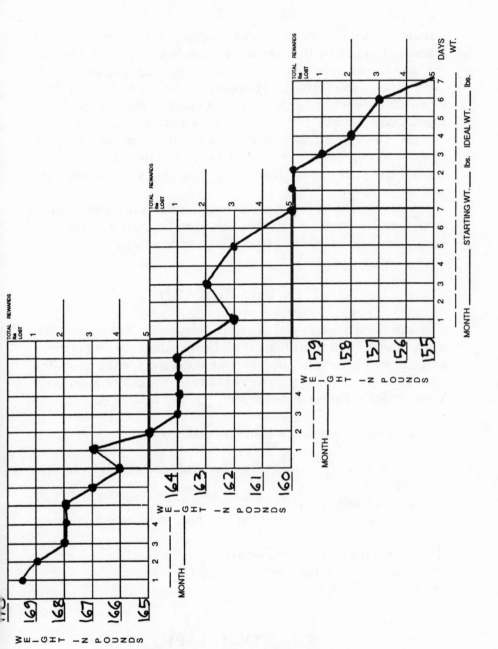

Milestones for Jack Taylor

but also notice that he yo-yoed a couple of times during Weeks 2 and 3. It's not easy to strike a perfect balance between the diet side and the exercise side of the fitness equation. You may inevitably suffer a few setbacks. However, if you maintain an overall downward direction with your own charts, you can use those momentary failures to spur you even more resolutely toward success. Once you reach your ideal weight, you can put your charts aside, or, better yet, you can tape them next to your representation of your ideal self, or next to photos of your formerly fat self.

Most of you wanting to shed from 5 to 50 pounds will fill out from 3 to 12 charts as you diet and exercise your way through your personalized 30- to 180-day starter programs.

THE BIG REWARD

Think of the day when you can store away your ideal representations, your Equilibrium Plan Slide Guide, and your calculations and charts. There you stand, looking good and feeling good. It's New Year's Eve, 1999, and you're ready to ring in a new century. What, exactly, have you achieved? The big reward of:

- An ideal weight and a lean fat-balanced body
- Radiant health
- A new level of high energy and full mental and physical capacity
- A higher idle speed
- The ability to eat more food and burn it off more quickly
- Low blood cholesterol
- Increased pride and self-respect
- An improved social life
- A longer life span

THE FINAL TAPE

As a professional ultra-athlete, I have competed in some of the toughest races in the world, from the Hawaiian Ironman Triathlon to the Western States 100-Mile Race. I love the long endurance events because they teach me so much about myself, forcing me to reach deep within me for energy, strength, and the will to continue.

When I look at my life and ask myself Who am I? I initially list the expected categories—author, businessperson, woman, journalist, athlete, editor, and friend—yet at my core I am an athlete first and foremost. But if I reach more deeply, asking myself Why? I always conclude, Because I want to feel alive in every cell of my body and every corner of my mind. This feeling of physical and mental aliveness strengthens my relationships with others and helps me climb to the top of my personal mountains. It helps me run when I'm ready to fall, it helps me pick myself up and dust myself off after I have fallen, and it makes me feel lucky and happy whenever I scamper or crawl across the finish line. We burst through many final tapes during our lifetimes, but only one of them will be truly final.

As I think ahead to the final tape of my physical and mental life, I imagine a sports stadium with a track surrounding a grassy field. I run into the stadium through a tunnel, much like the last few laps of the women's Olympic marathon. As I burst onto the track, I see the seats filled with my family and my friends. They smile and applaud. On the other side of the track I see the final tape and a fluttering banner beneath which stands a solitary figure.

In the center of the grass, I see a podium from which a judge recounts the story of my life. As I run, I realize that I alone wrote the script and that I alone made all the little and big decisions that ruled my life. As I round the first bend in the track, I hear the judge proclaim, "Sally was a good person. She was energetic, lived a full life, and helped and loved her friends."

When you imagine running toward your own final tape, what verdict does the judge render? What script have you been writing? What decisions about your physical and mental well-being have you been making?

As I round the last bend, I look up at the banner and see the inscription for the first time, "You Did Your Best," and I finally recognize that solitary figure beneath it: myself, the only one whose approval and congratulations for a life well lived ever really mattered.

APPENDIX

DIET AND EXERCISE CALORIES

The figures in these charts are based on averages. Considerable differences can occur among individual servings of foods and (in the case of exercise calories) among individuals. The author gratefully acknowledges the work of E. W. Bannister and S. R. Brown in "The Relative Energy Requirements of Physical Activities," which appeared in H. B. Falls, *Exercise Physiology* (New York: Academic Press, 1968).

Please note the following equivalents:

Weight		Volume	
1 ounce	=28.4 grams	1 tablespoon	=3 teaspoons
16 ounces		1 fluid ounce	=2 tablespoons
(one pound)	=454 grams	1 cup	=8 fluid ounces/
1 gram	=.035 ounce		one half pint
100 grams	=3.5 ounces		16 tablespoons
		1 quart	=4 cups

Job, exercise, and other activity calories are usually expressed, in the exercise physiology literature, as calories burned per minute. That is how they are expressed here. The Equilibrium Plan Slide Guide, on the other hand, expresses them as calories burned per half hour.

As explained in Chapter 2, food values are coded as follows:

CODE: ○ Good foods
    Nutritious, and 30 percent or less calories from fat
CODE: ■ Not-so-bad foods
    Nutritious but 30–60 percent calories from fat
CODE: × Bad foods
    Nonnutritious, or 60 percent or more calories from fat

MEAT AND FISH
NVF = no visible fat

Code		Calories	Fat, grams	% CALORIES FROM		
				Carbohydrates	Fat	Protein
■	Corned beef, 1 oz	61	3.4	—	52	48
■	Ground beef, 10% fat, 1 oz	62	3.2	—	48	52
×	Ground beef, 21% fat, 1 oz	81.2	6.2	—	67	33
■	Pot roast, NVF, 1 oz	54.6	2.5	—	39	61
■	Rib roast, NVF, 1 oz	68.3	3.8	—	52	48
■	Round steak, NVF, 1 oz	53.6	1.8	—	31	69
■	Sirloin steak, NVF, 1 oz	58.2	2	—	33	67
■	T-bone steak, NVF, 1 oz	63.4	2.9	—	43	57
■	Chicken breast, w/skin, 1 oz	55.8	2.2	—	37	63
○	Chicken breast, no skin, 1 oz	46.8	1	—	21	79
■	Leg w/skin, 1 oz	65.6	3.8	—	54	46
■	Drumstick, w/skin, 1 oz	61	3.2	—	48	52
■	Thigh, w/skin, 1 oz	70	4.4	—	58	42
■	Thigh, no skin, 1 oz	59	3.1	—	49	51
■	Wing, w/skin, 1 oz	82	5.5	—	62	38
○	Clams, steamed, 1 oz	24.8	0.46	13	17	70
○	Cod, steamed, 1 oz	23.7	0.26	—	10	90
×	Fish sticks, 1 piece	50	2.3	16	47	37
○	Halibut, steamed, 1 oz	37.4	1.1	—	27	73
○	Lobster, boiled, 1 oz	34	1	—	26	74
○	Oysters, raw, 1 oz	22.3	0.6	26	26	48
■	Salmon, steamed, 1 oz	56.2	3.7	—	59	41
■	Salmon, smoked, 1 oz	48.5	2.6	—	49	51
■	Salmon, canned, 1 oz	42.8	1.9	—	40	60
■	Sardines, drained, 1 oz	60.2	3.5	—	54	46
○	Scallops, steamed, 1 oz	30.8	0.43	12	11	76
×	Scampi, fried/frozen, 1 oz	90.2	5	36	49	15
○	Shrimp, boiled, 1 oz	33.4	0.7	—	18	82
○	Tuna, canned in water, 1 oz	36.2	0.23	—	6	94
×	Tuna salad, ½ cup	217	16.5	3	70	27
■	Lamb, NVF, 1 oz	61	3.2	—	48	52
■	Pork chop, NVF, 1 oz	70.3	4.1	—	52	48
×	Sausage link, 1	48	4	1	77	22
×	Bacon, 1 strip	36.3	3.1	29	56	15
■	Ham, NVF, 1 oz	44.3	1.5	—	33	67
×	Bologna, 1 slice	72	6.5	3	82	15

MEAT AND FISH *(Continued)*

Code		Calories	Fat, grams	% CALORIES FROM		
				Carbohydrates	Fat	Protein
✕	Hot dog, 1	183	16.6	3	83	14
○	Turkey, light meat, 1 oz	44.3	0.9	—	19	81
■	Turkey, dark meat, 1 oz	53	2	—	36	64
■	Veal cutlet, 1 oz	61.3	3.1	—	48	52
✕	Pâté, liver, 1 Tbs	41	3.6	2	80	18
■	Egg, 1 whole	79	5.6	3	65	32

DAIRY FOODS

Code		Calories	Fat, grams	% CALORIES FROM		
				Carbohydrates	Fat	Protein
×	Butter, 1 Tsp.	33.8	3.8	—	100	—
×	American cheese, 1 oz	106	8.5	2	74	24
×	Cheddar cheese, 1 oz	114	9.2	1	74	25
○	Cottage cheese, low-fat, ½ cup	102	2.2	17	20	63
×	Cottage cheese, ½ cup	109	4.5	11	39	50
■	Mozzarella cheese, part-skim, 1 oz	72	4.6	4	57	39
×	Neufchâtel cheese, 1 oz	74	6.7	4	81	15
■	Parmesan cheese, 1 Tbs	23	1.5	3	60	37
■	Ricotta cheese, part-skim, 1/3 cup	112	6.2	16	52	32
×	Ricotta cheese, regular, 1/3 cup	141	10.5	7	67	26
×	Cream, half and half, 1 Tbs	20	1.7	13	78	9
×	Whipped cream, ¼ cup	103	11.1	3	95	2
×	Sour cream, 1 Tbs	30.8	2.8	8	86	6
×	Nondairy topping, ¼ cup	60	4.7	28	70	2
×	Imitation sour cream, 1 Tbs	30	2.8	13	82	5

DAIRY FOODS *(Continued)*

Code		Calories	Fat, grams	% CALORIES FROM		
				Carbohydrates	Fat	Protein
○	Nonfat dry milk, 1 Tbs	15.2	0.03	59	2	39
✕	Margarine, 1 Tsp	34	3.8	—	100	—
■	Milk, whole, 1 cup	150	8	30	49	21
■	Milk, 2%, low-fat, 1 cup	121	4.8	38	35	27
○	Milk, skim, 1 cup	86	0.44	56	5	39
✕	Hot cocoa, 1 cup	218	10.1	45	39	16
✕	Ice cream, regular, 1 cup	269	15.4	44	49	7
✕	Ice cream, rich, 1 cup	349	23.7	35	60	5
○	Ice milk, 1 cup	184	5.6	62	27	11
✕	Pudding, 1 cup	320	7.8	69	21	10
✕	Sherbet, 1 cup	270	3.8	85	12	3
○	Yogurt, nonfat, plain, 1 cup	about 90	less than 1	53	7	40
○	Yogurt, low-fat, plain, 1 cup	144	3.4	45	22	33
■	Yogurt, low-fat, flavored, 1 cup	231	2.4	74	9	17
○	Yogurt, nonfat, flavored, 1 cup	about 150	less than 1	72	4	24

FRUITS AND NUTS

Code		Calories	Fat, grams	% CALORIES FROM		
				Carbohydrates	Fat	Protein
O	Apple, 1	81	0.5	94	5	1
O	juice, 1 cup	111	0.25	97	2	1
O	sauce, ½ cup	53	0.06	98	1	1
O	Apricots, 3 fresh	51	0.41	83	7	10
O	juice-packed, ½ cup	59.5	0.045	94	1	5
X	Avocado, medium	324	30	11	83	6
O	Banana, 1	105	0.55	92	4	4
O	Blackberries, ½ cup	37	0.28	89	6	5
O	Blueberries, ½ cup	41	0.27	90	6	4
O	Boysenberries, ½ cup	33	0.175	88	4	8
O	Cherries, 1 cup	104	1.4	83	11	6
O	Dates, 5	114	0.19	96	1	3
O	Fruit cocktail, juice-packed, ½ cup	56.6	0.015	96	0	4
O	Grapefruit, 1 whole	79	0.24	90	3	7
O	Grapefruit juice, 1 cup	96	0.25	93	2	5
O	Grapes, 1 cup	114	0.92	90	7	3
O	Grape juice, 1 cup	128	0.23	97	2	1
O	Kiwi, 1 whole	46	0.34	88	6	6
O	Mandarin orange, ½ cup	70	0.05	95	1	4
O	Melon, cantaloupe, 1 cup	48	0.44	81	8	11
O	Melon, honeydew, 1 cup	60	0.17	93	2	5
O	Watermelon, 1 cup	50	0.68	82	11	7
O	Nectarine slices, 1 cup	68	0.63	86	7	7
O	Orange, 1 whole	62	0.16	91	2	7
O	Orange juice, 1 cup	111	0.5	90	4	6
O	Peach, 1 whole	37	0.08	92	2	6
O	juice-packed, 1 cup	109	0.08	94	1	5
O	Pear, 1 whole	98	0.66	93	5	2
O	juice-packed, 1 cup	123	0.16	96	1	3
O	Pineapple, juice-packed, ½ cup	75	0.1	96	1	3
O	Pineapple juice, 1 cup	139	0.2	97	1	2
O	Plums, 2 whole	72	0.82	86	9	5
O	Prunes, 2 whole	40.2	0.085	94	2	4
O	Raisins, ¼ cup	124	0.19	95	1	4
O	Raspberries, ½ cup	30.5	0.34	84	9	7
O	Strawberries, 1 cup	45	0.55	83	10	7
O	Tangerine, 1 whole	37	0.16	92	3	5
X	Almonds, roasted, ¼ cup	246	22.6	12	77	11
X	Cashews, roasted, ¼ cup	196	15.9	19	69	12

FRUITS AND NUTS *(Continued)*

Code		Calories	Fat, grams	% CALORIES FROM		
				Carbohydrates	Fat	Protein
✕	Peanuts, roasted, ¼ cup	210	17.9	11	73	16
✕	Peanut butter, ⅛ cup	185	16	10	74	16
✕	Sunflower seeds, dry, ¼ cup	203	17.1	13	71	16
✕	Walnuts, English, chopped, 1 Tbs	49	4.8	9	83	8

BREADS AND CEREALS

Code		Calories	Fat, grams	% CALORIES FROM Carbohydrates	Fat	Protein
O	Corn grits, 1 cup	146	0.5	87	3	10
O	Oats, cooked, 1 cup	145	2.4	69	15	16
O	Popcorn, plain, 1 cup	23	0.3	76	11	13
O	Rice, brown, 1 cup cooked	232	1.6	86	6	8
O	Rice, white, 1 cup cooked	237	0.51	91	2	7
O	Wheat germ, plain, 1 Tbs	27	0.8	48	24	28
O	Bagel, 1	255	1	78	6	16
O	Cornbread muffin, 1	130	4.2	62	29	9
O	Dry bread cubes, ¼ cup	27.7	0.3	77	9	14
O	White bread, 1 slice	75	0.9	76	11	13
O	Whole-wheat bread, 1 slice	65	0.7	77	9	14
X	Brownie, from bakery, 1	86	4	56	40	4
X	Cheesecake, 3.8 oz	269	18.7	32	63	5
X	Chocolate cake, 2.4 oz	234	8.5	64	31	5
X	Coffee cake, 2″ square	232	7	65	27	8
O	Cereal, high-fiber type, 1 cup	150	1	83	7	10
■	Cereal, high-sugar type, 1 cup	146	2.9	77	18	5
■	Oats, instant packet, 1 cup	154	1.8	78	10	12
X	Chocolate-chip cookie, homemade, 1	108	6.3	44	51	5
X	Oatmeal-raisin cookie, 1	58.7	2	64	31	5
X	Peanut-butter cookie, 1	95	5.8	37	54	9
X	Sandwich-type cookie, 1	49.5	2.2	56	40	4
■	Corn tortilla, no fat, 1	63	3	62	31	7
X	Tortilla chips, 2 oz	278	15	47	47	6
X	Cheese cracker, 1	5.2	0.23	50	41	9
X	Ritz cracker, 1	18	1	47	48	5
X	Saltine cracker, 1	12	0.33	67	25	8
■	Saltine thin cracker, 1	9	0.35	58	36	6
X	Croissant, 6″ long, 1	246	13	44	48	8
X	Doughnut, cake-type, 1	98	4.7	52	43	5
X	Doughnut, yeast-type, 1	176	11	36	58	6
X	Cheese puffs, 2 oz	316	19.6	37	57	6
X	Potato chips, 2 oz	326	22.6	34	62	4
O	Pretzels, 2 oz	221	2.5	79	11	10
X	Eclair, 1	240	13.6	39	51	10
■	Graham cracker, 1	27.5	0.65	72	20	8
O	Blueberry muffin, 1	112	3.7	60	30	10

BREADS AND CEREALS *(Continued)*

Code		Calories	Fat, grams	% CALORIES FROM		
				Carbohydrates	Fat	Protein
○	Bran muffin, 1	105	3.9	59	30	11
■	Crepe, no filling, 1	58	2.6	45	41	14
○	Pancake, mix, 1	70	2	58	30	12
○	Spaghetti, 1 cup cooked	172	0.7	82	4	14
×	Danish pastry, 1	274	15.3	43	50	7
×	Poptart, 1	200	5	72	22	6
×	Twinkie, 1	186	10	46	48	6
×	Fruit pie, 4.6 oz	403	17.5	59	38	3
×	Cream-type pie, 4.6 oz	384	22.4	38	52	10
■	Waffles, mix, one 9″ square	206	8	53	34	13
○	Waffles, frozen, one 4″ square	86	2.1	67	22	11

VEGETABLES

Code		Calories	Fat, grams	% CALORIES FROM		
				Carbohydrates	Fat	Protein
O	Alfalfa sprouts, ¼ cup	2.5	0.06	40	17	43
O	Artichoke, 1 whole	31.5	0.2	76	3	21
O	Asparagus, 1 cup	29	0.3	57	7	36
O	Bean sprouts, 1/3 cup	14.8	0.07	61	4	35
O	Garbanzo beans, ¼ cup	62.5	1.1	63	16	21
O	Kidney beans, ¼ cup	56.5	0.24	70	4	26
O	Pinto beans, ½ cup	125	0.5	73	4	23
O	Refried beans, ½ cup	123	3.33	52	24	24
O	Broccoli, 1 cup	34	0.5	44	11	45
O	Brussels sprouts, 1 cup	42	0.6	48	10	42
O	Cabbage, 1 cup cooked	25.5	0.3	64	9	27
O	Carrot, 1 raw	25.3	0.13	86	4	10
O	Cauliflower, 1 cup cooked	19.5	0.3	49	11	40
O	Celery, 6" stalk	5	0.03	71	5	24
O	Greens, 1 cup cooked	63	1.3	50	15	35
O	Corn, 1 cup	130	1.05	82	6	12
O	Cucumber, diced, ¼ cup	5.3	0.04	74	5	21
O	Eggplant, ½ cup	19	0.2	74	8	18
O	Green peas, ½ cup	49.5	0.31	62	5	33
O	Green peppers, raw, ¼ cup	7.5	0.1	64	12	24
O	Lettuce, iceberg, 1 cup	6.8	0.16	55	17	28
O	Lettuce, romaine, 1 cup	10	0.21	49	21	30
O	Mushrooms, raw, ¼ cup sliced	3.7	0.08	55	14	41
X	Olives, black, 5 whole	39	4.7	5	93	2
O	Black-eyed peas, ½ cup	95	0.4	70	4	26
O	Potato, 1 whole	145	0.2	88	1	11
O	Potatoes, hash browns, ½ cup	173	8.9	51	45	4
O	Potatoes, mashed, 1 cup	135	1.5	78	10	12
O	Spinach, raw, 3½ oz.	26	0.3	66	10	24
O	Spinach, cooked, 1 cup	40	1.0	66	10	24
O	Summer squash, 1 cup	29	0.2	73	5	22
O	Winter squash, 1 cup	91	0.7	83	6	11
O	Sweet potato, 1 whole	160	0.75	90	4	6
■	Tofu, 1 piece (2½" × 2¼" × 1")	86	5	12	48	40
O	Tomatoes, ½ cup	39	0.4	78	8	14
O	Tomato juice, 1 cup	45	0.24	80	4	16
O	Tomato, raw, 1 whole	25	0.2	81	6	13

CONVENIENCE FOODS

Code		Calories	Fat, grams	% CALORIES FROM		
				Carbohydrates	Fat	Protein
✕	Cheese soufflé, 1 cup	301	23.1	11	70	19
✕	Chicken pot pie, 1 whole	430	23	38	48	14
■	Chili, 1 cup	339	15.6	36	41	23
✕	Chocolate mousse, ¾ cup	250	10.1	53	35	12
✕	Gelatin dessert, ¾ cup	107	—	90	—	10
✕	Popsicle, 1	70	—	100	—	—
■	Beef/vegetable stew, homemade, 1 cup	225	8.5	24	33	43
■	Meatloaf, beef, baked, 2.25 oz, 1 slice	200	8.8	19	40	41
■	Macaroni and cheese, homemade, 1 cup	293	10.8	53	33	14
■	Manicotti w/meat and cheese, homemade, 1 each	390	20	26	46	28
	Kentucky Fried Chicken (original recipe)					
✕	Wing, 1, with skin	136	9	12	59	29
■	Drumstick, 1, with skin	117	6.5	9	50	41
■	Breast, 1, with skin	236	12.3	12	47	41
✕	Thigh, 1, with skin	257	17.5	10	61	29
✕	Coleslaw, 1 serving	121	7.5	42	55	3
○	Ear of corn, 1 serving	169	2.8	74	15	11
○	Mashed potatoes, 1 serving	63.9	0.9	79	13	10
✕	Gravy, 1 serving	22.7	1.8	23	70	7
	McDonald's					
■	Egg McMuffin, 1	327	14.8	37	41	22
○	English muffin with butter, 1	186	5.3	64	26	10
✕	Hash browns, 1 serving	125	7	45	50	5
■	Hot cakes with butter and syrup, 1 serving	500	10.3	75	19	6
✕	Sausage, 1 serving	206	18.6	1	82	17
✕	Scrambled eggs, 1 serving	180	13	6	65	29
✕	Big Mac, 1	563	33	29	53	18
■	Cheese burger, 1 serving	307	14.1	39	41	20
✕	Chicken McNuggets, 6-piece order	314	19	20	54	26
✕	Filet O'Fish, 1 serving	432	25	35	52	13

CONVENIENCE FOODS (Continued)

Code		Calories	Fat, grams	% CALORIES FROM		
				Carbohydrates	Fat	Protein
✕	French fries (2.8 oz) 1 serving	220	11.5	47	47	5
▪	Hamburger, 1	255	9.8	46	35	19
▪	Milkshake, chocolate, 1 serving	383	9	68	21	10
✕	Quarter Pounder with cheese, 1	524	30.7	25	53	23
▪	Quarter Pounder, 1	424	21.7	31	46	23
✕	Chocolate-chip cookies, 1 package	342	16.3	52	43	5
✕	Pie, apple, fried, 1	253	14.3	46	51	3
	Mexican Type					
○	Bean burrito, 1 serving	343	12	56	31	13
▪	Combination burrito, 1 serving	404	16	43	36	21
▪	Beef enchilada, 1 serving	317	20.8	26	56	18
▪	Chicken enchilada, 1 serving	247	14	33	48	19
▪	Cheese enchilada, 1 serving	318	19.5	28	53	19
▪	Beef taco, 1	192	11	23	52	25
▪	Chicken taco, 1	157	7.2	22	41	37
○	Tostada, bean, 1 serving	180	6	53	28	19
▪	Tostada, beef and bean, 1 serving	239	14.4	28	53	20
▪	Tostada, chicken and bean, 1 serving	214	10.5	31	44	25
✕	Onion rings, 1 serving	284	16	44	51	6
✕	Corn dog, 1	330	20	33	55	12
▪	Cheese pizza (⅛ of 14″), 1 slice	232	8.7	46	34	20
✕	Quiche (1/7th of 9″ diameter pie)	391	25.4	25	57	18
✕	Chicken salad, ½ cup	264	20.8	3	71	76
✕	Macaroni salad, ½ cup	179	13.6	24	74	2
✕	Egg salad, ½ cup	314	30.5	2	87	11
✕	Potato salad, ½ cup	195	14.6	26	67	7
	Salad Dressings					
✕	Blue cheese, regular, 1 Tbs	77	8	6	91	4

CONVENIENCE FOODS *(Continued)*

Code		Calories	Fat, grams	% CALORIES FROM		
				Carbohydrates	Fat	Protein
×	Italian, regular, 1 Tbs	68.6	7.12	9	91	1
×	Thousand Island, regular, 1 Tbs	58.9	5.6	16	83	1
×	Italian, low-calorie, 1 Tbs	15.8	1.47	18	82	—
×	Thousand Island, low-calorie, 1 Tbs	24.3	1.6	40	59	2
	Soups					
○	Chicken noodle, 1 cup	75	2.4	49	29	21
■	Clam chowder, New England, 1 cup	163	6.6	41	36	23
○	Clam chowder, Manhattan, 1 cup	78	2.3	57	24	19
×	Cream of mushroom, 1 cup	203	13.6	29	59	12
○	Minestrone, 1 cup	83	2.5	53	27	20
■	Spaghetti sauce with meat, ½ cup	149	9.2	26	54	20
■	Spaghetti sauce, meatless, ½ cup	91.3	4.8	47	44	8

SAUCES, BEVERAGES, AND CANDY

Code		Calories	Fat, grams	% CALORIES FROM		
				Carbohydrates	Fat	Protein
×	Gravy, beef, with white flour, ¼ cup	75.5	6.5	16	78	6
×	White sauce, ¼ cup	95.5	6.9	25	65	10
×	Barbecue sauce, 1 Tbs	14.2	1.08	32	62	6
×	Ketchup, 1 Tbs	18.1	0.07	90	3	7
×	Mayonnaise, 1 Tbs	32.8	3.6	1	98	1
■	Mustard, 1 Tbs	3.9	0.23	30	47	22
×	Tartar sauce, 1 Tbs	74	8.1	3	96	1
×	Honey, 1 Tbs	21.4	—	100	—	—
×	Jam, 1 Tbs	54	0.02	99	—	1
×	Syrup, maple, 1 Tbs	51	—	100	—	—
×	Sugar, white, 1 Tsp	16	—	100	—	—
×	Chocolate fudge topping, 2 Tbs	104	4.0	60	35	5
	Beverages					
×	Fruit soda, 12 oz	156	—	100	—	—
×	Kool-Aid with sugar, 12 oz	142	—	100	—	—
×	Cola-type soda, 12 oz	136	—	100	—	—
×	Beer, 12 oz	143	—	93	—	7
×	Wine, 8 oz	151	—	86	1	14
×	Hard liquor, 1½ oz	106	—	100	—	—
	Candy					
×	Fudge, 1 oz	114	4.9	61	36	3
×	Hard candy, 1 oz	109	0.3	98	2	—
×	Jelly candy, 1 oz	98	0.2	98	2	0
×	M&M's, peanut, 1 oz	145	7.3	46	45	9
×	Milk chocolate, plain, 1 oz	147	9.2	41	53	6
×	Snickers, 1 oz	138	6.5	49	43	9
×	Reese's peanut butter cups, 1 cup	120	7.2	37	54	10

JOB CALORIES PER MINUTE

Job	110	130	150	170	190	210
	WEIGHT (POUNDS)					
Assembly-line work/light	2.9	3.3	3.7	4.1	4.5	4.9
Baking	1.8	2.1	2.4	2.7	3.0	3.3
Bartending (busy)	3.0	3.4	3.8	4.2	4.6	5.0
Carpentry	2.6	3.1	3.5	4.0	4.5	4.9
Cash register operator	1.8	2.0	2.2	2.4	2.6	2.8
Cooking (F)	2.3	2.7	3.1	3.5	3.9	4.3
Cooking (M)	2.4	2.8	3.3	3.7	4.1	4.6
Counseling	2.3	2.7	3.1	3.5	3.9	4.3
Delivery service	1.8	2.1	2.4	2.7	3.0	3.3
Driving (active)	3.0	3.4	3.8	4.2	4.6	5.0
Electrical work	2.9	3.4	3.9	4.5	5.0	5.5
Farming						
feeding animals	3.3	3.8	4.4	5.0	5.6	6.2
milking by hand	2.7	3.2	3.7	4.2	4.6	5.1
Forestry						
ax-chopping, fast	14.9	17.5	20.2	22.9	25.5	28.2
hoeing	4.6	5.4	6.2	7.0	7.8	8.6
stacking firewood	4.4	5.2	6.0	6.8	7.6	8.4
weeding	3.6	4.2	4.9	5.5	6.2	6.8
Gas-station attendant	3.3	3.7	4.1	4.5	4.9	5.4
Housewife/househusband	3.3	3.7	4.1	4.5	4.9	5.4
Keyboarding	1.9	2.1	2.3	2.5	2.7	2.9
Lab technician	2.9	3.3	3.7	4.1	4.5	4.9
Machine tooling						
operating lathe	2.6	3.1	3.5	4.0	4.5	4.9
welding	2.6	3.1	3.5	4.0	4.5	4.9
Managerial (desk)	3.0	3.4	3.8	4.2	4.6	5.0
Managerial (active)	3.3	3.7	4.1	4.5	4.9	5.4
Mechanic	3.3	3.7	4.1	4.5	4.9	5.4
Nursing care	2.7	3.2	3.7	4.2	4.6	5.1
Painting, inside	1.7	2.0	2.3	2.6	2.9	3.2
Painting, outside	3.9	4.5	5.2	5.9	6.6	7.3
Phoning (active)	2.9	3.3	3.7	4.1	4.5	4.9
Retail (light)	1.8	2.1	2.4	2.7	3.0	3.3
Retail (active)	3.0	3.4	3.8	4.2	4.6	5.0
Secretary/office work	1.9	2.1	2.3	2.5	2.7	2.9
Stewardess/airlines	3.0	3.4	3.8	4.2	4.6	5.0
Tailoring						
hand sewing	1.6	1.9	2.2	2.5	2.8	3.0
pressing	3.1	3.7	4.2	4.8	5.3	5.9
Teaching	3.0	3.4	3.8	4.2	4.6	5.0
Traveling sales	2.7	3.2	3.7	4.2	4.6	5.1
Waiting tables	3.0	3.4	3.8	4.2	4.6	5.0
Window cleaning (F)	3.0	3.5	4.0	4.5	5.1	5.6

JOB CALORIES PER MINUTE *(Continued)*

Job	WEIGHT (POUNDS)					
	110	130	150	170	190	210
Window cleaning (M)	2.9	3.4	3.9	4.5	5.0	5.5
Writing (sitting)	1.5	1.7	2.0	2.2	2.5	2.8

EXERCISE CALORIES PER MINUTE

Activity	110	130	150	170	190	210
	BODY WEIGHT (POUNDS)					
Archery	4.0	4.6	5.2	5.8	6.4	7.0
Badminton						
recreational, singles	4.6	5.2	5.8	6.4	7.0	7.6
recreational, doubles	3.9	4.5	5.1	5.7	6.3	6.9
competitive, doubles	6.0	6.8	7.6	8.4	9.2	10.0
competitive, singles	8.0	9.1	10.2	11.3	12.4	13.5
Baseball						
other than pitcher or catcher	3.7	4.2	4.7	5.2	5.7	6.2
pitcher only	5.1	5.8	6.5	7.2	7.9	8.6
catcher only	4.5	5.2	5.9	6.6	7.3	8.0
Basketball						
nongame, half court, etc.	7.3	8.3	9.3	10.3	11.3	12.3
officiating	7.3	8.3	9.3	10.3	11.3	12.3
game (full court, cont.)	9.8	11.2	12.6	14.0	15.4	16.8
Bench stepping, 30 steps per minute						
7"	8.5	9.6	10.7	11.8	12.9	14.0
12"	10.4	11.9	13.4	14.9	16.4	17.9
16"	14.5	16.5	18.5	20.5	22.5	24.5
18"	18.3	20.8	23.3	25.8	28.3	30.5
Bicycling						
5½ mph	3.2	3.6	4.0	4.4	4.8	5.2
10 mph	5.4	6.2	7.0	7.8	8.6	9.4
13 mph	8.6	9.8	11.0	12.2	13.4	14.6
Bowling						
continuous	3.5	4.0	4.5	5.0	5.5	6.0
regular	2.5	2.9	3.3	3.7	4.1	4.5
Calisthenics, general	3.9	4.5	5.1	5.7	6.3	6.9
Canoeing						
2 mph	3.9	4.5	5.1	5.7	6.3	6.9
4 mph	8.2	9.3	10.4	11.5	12.6	13.7
Dancing						
aerobic (low)	3.4	4.1	4.8	5.5	6.2	6.9
aerobic (medium)	5.8	6.6	7.4	8.2	9.0	9.8
aerobic (high)	8.6	9.8	11.0	12.2	13.4	14.6
fox trot	3.3	3.8	4.3	4.8	5.3	5.8
contemporary (rock)	3.3	3.8	4.3	4.8	5.3	5.8
waltz	3.3	3.8	4.3	4.8	5.3	5.8
rumba	3.9	4.5	5.1	5.7	6.3	6.9
square	5.5	6.3	7.1	7.9	8.7	9.5
polka	6.5	7.4	8.3	9.2	10.1	11.0

EXERCISE CALORIES PER MINUTE *(Continued)*

Activity	BODY WEIGHT (POUNDS)					
	110	130	150	170	190	210
Fencing						
recreational	3.9	4.5	5.1	5.7	6.3	6.9
competitive (vigorous)	8.0	9.1	10.2	11.3	12.4	13.5
Fishing						
boat	1.8	2.0	2.2	2.4	2.6	2.8
ice	2.3	3.0	3.7	4.4	5.1	5.8
standing (little movement)	2.0	2.4	2.8	5.2	5.6	6.0
surf	2.3	2.7	3.1	3.5	3.9	4.3
stream, wading	3.9	4.5	5.1	5.7	6.3	6.9
Football						
playground (touch)	7.8	8.9	10.1	11.2	12.3	13.4
officiating	7.3	8.3	9.3	10.3	11.3	12.3
tackle	11.0	12.5	14.0	15.5	17.0	17.5
Golf						
foursome 9 holes in 2 hr (carry clubs)	3.5	4.0	4.5	5.0	5.5	6.0
foursome 9 holes in 2 hr (pull clubs)	3.3	3.8	4.3	4.8	5.3	5.8
cart	2.9	3.3	3.7	4.1	4.5	4.9
driving	3.3	3.8	4.3	4.8	5.3	5.8
putting	2.0	2.3	2.6	2.9	3.2	3.5
twosome 9 holes in 1½ hr (carrying clubs)	4.9	5.7	6.5	7.3	8.1	8.9
twosome 9 holes in 1½ hr (pull clubs)	4.3	4.9	5.5	6.1	6.7	7.3
Gymnastics						
light	3.9	4.5	5.1	5.7	6.3	6.9
medium	6.7	7.6	8.5	9.4	10.3	11.2
hard	9.3	10.6	11.9	13.2	14.5	15.8
Handball						
cutthroat	7.8	8.9	9.0	10.1	11.2	12.3
doubles	6.7	7.6	8.5	9.4	10.3	11.2
singles	10.2	11.6	13.0	14.4	15.8	17.2
Hiking						
20-lb pack, 2 mph	3.9	4.5	5.1	5.7	6.3	6.9
20-lb pack, 3½ mph	5.0	5.7	6.4	7.1	7.8	8.5
20-lb pack, 4 mph	5.9	6.7	7.5	8.3	9.1	9.9
Hill climbing	7.8	8.9	10.0	11.1	12.2	13.3
Hockey						
ice	11.8	13.4	15.0	16.6	17.2	18.8
field	11.8	13.4	15.0	16.6	17.2	18.8
Horseback riding						
walk	2.2	2.5	2.8	3.1	3.4	3.7

EXERCISE CALORIES PER MINUTE *(Continued)*

Activity	BODY WEIGHT (POUNDS)					
	110	130	150	170	190	210
trot	5.4	6.2	7.0	7.8	8.6	9.4
gallop	7.8	8.9	10.0	11.1	12.2	13.3
Horseshoes	3.0	3.4	3.8	4.2	4.6	5.0
Isometrics	3.0	3.4	3.8	4.2	4.6	5.0
Judo	10.3	11.8	13.3	14.8	16.3	17.8
Karate	10.3	11.8	13.3	14.8	16.3	17.8
Lacrosse	11.8	13.4	15.0	16.6	17.2	18.8
Martial arts	10.3	11.8	13.3	14.8	16.3	17.8
Mountain climbing	7.8	8.9	10.0	11.1	12.2	13.3
Orienteering	7.8	8.9	10.0	11.1	12.2	13.3
Rope skipping						
alternate feet, 50–60 per minute each foot	6.7	7.6	8.5	9.4	10.3	11.2
alternate feet, 70–80 per minute each foot	7.3	8.3	9.3	10.3	11.3	12.3
alternate feet, 90–100 per minute each foot	8.6	9.8	11.0	12.2	13.4	14.6
alternate feet, 110–120 per minute each foot	11.8	13.4	15.0	16.6	17.2	18.8
alternate feet, 130–140 per minute each foot	15.7	17.8	19.9	22.0	24.1	26.2
Rowing						
pleasure, 2 mph	3.9	4.5	5.1	5.7	6.3	6.9
vigorous, 4 mph	8.6	9.8	11.0	12.2	13.4	13.6
Rowing machine						
easy	3.9	4.5	5.1	5.7	6.3	6.9
vigorous	8.6	9.8	11.0	12.2	13.4	13.6
Run in place						
50–60 steps per min (left foot only)	6.7	7.6	8.5	9.4	10.3	11.2
70–80 steps per min (left foot only)	7.3	8.3	9.3	10.3	11.3	12.3
90–100 steps per min (left foot only)	8.6	9.8	11.0	12.2	13.4	14.6
110–120 steps per min (left foot only)	11.8	13.4	15.0	16.6	17.2	18.8
130–140 steps per min (left foot only)	15.7	17.8	19.9	22.0	24.1	26.2
Running						
5.5 mph	8.6	9.8	11.0	12.2	13.4	14.6
6.0 mph	8.8	9.9	11.0	12.1	13.2	14.3
6.5 mph	8.9	10.2	11.5	12.8	14.1	15.4
7.0 mph	9.2	10.4	11.6	12.8	14.0	15.2

EXERCISE CALORIES PER MINUTE *(Continued)*

Activity	BODY WEIGHT (POUNDS)					
	110	130	150	170	190	210
7.5 mph	9.8	11.2	13.6	16.0	18.4	19.8
8.0 mph	10.4	11.9	13.4	14.9	16.4	17.9
8.5 mph	11.2	12.8	14.4	16.0	17.6	19.2
9.0 mph	12.0	13.8	15.6	17.4	19.2	21.0
9.5 mph	12.8	14.7	16.6	18.5	20.4	22.3
10.0 mph	13.6	15.5	17.4	19.3	21.2	23.1
10.5 mph	14.3	16.3	18.3	20.3	22.4	24.3
11.0 mph	15.2	17.3	19.4	21.5	23.7	25.9
11.5 mph	15.9	18.2	20.5	22.8	25.1	27.4
12.0 mph	18.2	20.7	23.2	25.7	28.2	30.7
12.5 mph	20.3	23.1	25.9	28.7	31.5	34.3
Sailing						
calm water	2.0	2.3	2.6	2.9	3.2	3.5
rough water	2.4	2.8	3.2	3.6	4.0	4.4
Scuba diving	5.9	6.7	7.5	8.3	9.1	10.0
Sprinting	31.9	36.3	40.7	45.1	49.5	53.9
Skating (leisure)						
ice	4.6	5.2	5.8	6.4	7.0	7.6
roller	4.6	5.2	5.8	6.4	7.0	7.6
Skating (vigorous)						
ice	8.1	9.3	10.5	11.7	12.9	14.1
roller	8.1	9.3	10.5	11.7	12.9	14.1
Skiing						
downhill (continuous, riding and lifts not included)	7.8	8.8	9.8	10.8	11.8	12.8
cross country, 5 mph	9.2	10.4	11.6	12.8	14.0	15.2
cross country, 9 mph	13.1	14.9	16.7	18.5	20.3	22.1
Skin diving	5.9	6.7	7.5	8.3	9.1	9.9
Sledding	5.6	6.3	7.0	7.7	8.5	9.2
Snowshoeing, 2.2 mph	5.0	5.7	6.4	7.1	7.8	8.5
Soccer	7.8	8.9	10.0	11.1	12.2	13.3
Stationary bicycle (resistance sufficient to get pulse rate to 130)						
10 mph	5.5	6.3	7.1	7.9	8.7	9.5
15 mph	8.6	9.8	11.0	12.2	13.4	14.6
20 mph	11.7	13.3	14.9	16.5	18.1	19.7
Swimming (crawl)						
20 yd per min	3.9	4.5	5.1	5.7	6.3	6.9
30 yd per min	5.5	6.3	7.1	7.9	9.7	10.5
35 yd per min	7.1	8.0	8.9	9.8	10.7	11.6
40 yd per min	7.8	8.9	10.0	11.1	12.2	13.3
45 yd per min	9.0	10.3	11.6	12.9	14.2	15.5

EXERCISE CALORIES PER MINUTE *(Continued)*

Activity	BODY WEIGHT (POUNDS)					
	110	130	150	170	190	210
55 yd per min	11.0	12.5	14.0	15.5	17.0	18.5
Table tennis						
recreational	3.9	4.5	5.1	5.7	6.3	6.9
vigorous	5.9	6.7	7.5	8.3	9.1	9.9
Tennis (singles)						
recreational	5.6	6.3	7.0	7.7	8.5	9.2
competitive	7.8	8.9	10.0	11.1	12.2	13.3
Tennis (doubles)						
recreational	3.9	4.5	5.1	5.7	6.3	6.9
competitive	5.6	6.3	7.0	7.7	8.5	9.2
Trampolining	10.3	11.8	13.3	14.8	16.3	17.8
Volleyball						
recreational	4.6	5.2	5.8	6.4	7.0	7.6
competitive	7.8	8.9	10.0	11.1	12.2	13.3
Walking						
2 mph	2.4	2.8	3.2	3.6	4.0	4.4
2.5 mph	3.3	3.8	4.3	4.8	5.3	5.8
3 mph	3.9	4.5	5.1	5.7	6.3	6.9
3.5 mph	4.1	4.7	5.3	5.9	6.5	7.1
4 mph	4.5	5.2	5.9	6.6	7.3	8.0
4.5 mph	5.9	6.7	7.5	8.3	9.1	9.9
5 mph	7.3	8.3	9.3	10.3	11.3	12.3
5.5 mph	8.6	9.8	11.0	12.2	13.4	14.6
upstairs normal	5.9	6.7	7.5	8.3	9.1	9.9
downstairs normal	5.9	6.7	7.5	8.3	9.1	9.9
upstairs, two at a time, rapidly	8.7	14.8	20.9	27.0	33.1	39.2
Weight training	3.9	4.5	5.1	5.7	6.3	6.9
Yoga	3.0	3.4	3.8	4.2	4.6	5.0

This weight-adjusted calories chart is based on averages. Considerable differences occur among individuals.

OTHER DAILY CALORIES PER MINUTE

Activity	BODY WEIGHT (POUNDS)					
	110	130	150	170	190	210
Card playing	1.3	1.5	1.7	1.9	2.2	2.4
Carpet sweeping (F)	2.3	2.7	3.1	3.5	3.9	4.3
Carpet sweeping (M)	2.4	2.8	3.3	3.7	4.1	4.6
Cleaning (F)	3.1	3.7	4.2	4.8	5.3	5.9
Cleaning (M)	2.9	3.4	3.9	4.5	5.0	5.5
Cooking/dinner	1.7	2.0	2.3	2.6	2.9	3.2
Driving car, automatic	1.3	1.4	1.5	1.6	1.7	1.8
Eating	1.3	1.4	1.5	1.6	1.7	1.8
Food shopping (F)	3.1	3.7	4.2	4.8	5.3	5.9
Food shopping (M)	2.9	3.4	3.9	4.5	5.0	5.5
Gardening						
digging	6.3	7.4	8.6	9.7	10.5	12.0
hedging	3.9	4.5	5.2	5.9	6.6	7.3
mowing	5.6	6.6	7.6	8.6	9.6	10.6
raking	2.7	3.2	3.7	4.2	4.6	5.1
Horse grooming	6.4	7.6	8.7	9.9	11.0	12.2
Ironing (F)	1.7	1.9	2.2	2.5	2.8	3.1
Ironing (M)	3.2	3.8	4.4	4.9	5.5	6.1
Knitting, sewing (F)	1.1	1.3	1.5	1.7	1.9	2.1
Knitting, sewing (M)	1.2	1.4	1.6	1.8	2.0	2.2
Making beds	2.7	3.1	3.5	3.9	4.3	4.7
Mopping floor (F)	3.1	3.7	4.2	4.8	5.3	5.9
Mopping floor (M)	2.9	3.4	3.9	4.5	5.0	5.5
Moving furniture	2.6	3.0	3.4	3.8	4.2	4.6
Music playing						
accordion	1.6	1.9	2.2	2.5	2.8	3.0
conducting	2.0	2.3	2.7	3.0	3.4	3.7
drums	3.3	3.9	4.5	5.1	5.7	6.3
horn	1.5	1.7	2.0	2.2	2.5	2.8
organ	2.7	3.1	3.6	4.1	4.6	5.0
piano	2.0	2.4	2.7	3.1	3.4	3.8
violin	2.3	2.7	3.1	3.5	3.9	4.3
Sawing, power	3.0	3.4	3.8	4.2	4.6	5.0
Scraping paint	3.2	3.7	4.3	4.9	5.4	6.0
Scrubbing floors (F)	5.5	6.4	7.4	8.4	9.4	10.4
Scrubbing floors (M)	5.4	6.4	7.3	8.3	9.3	10.3
Sex						
intercourse	4.0	4.5	5.0	5.5	6.0	6.5
foreplay	1.8	2.0	2.2	2.4	2.6	2.8
Showering and dressing	2.6	3.0	3.4	3.8	4.2	4.6
Sitting quietly	1.1	1.2	1.4	1.6	1.8	2.0
Sitting talking	1.3	1.5	1.7	1.9	2.2	2.4
Sleeping	0.9	1.0	1.1	1.2	1.3	1.4

OTHER DAILY CALORIES PER MINUTE *(Continued)*

Activity	BODY WEIGHT (POUNDS)					
	110	130	150	170	190	210
Standing quietly (F)	1.3	1.5	1.7	1.9	2.2	2.4
Standing quietly (M)	1.4	1.6	1.8	2.2	2.4	2.6
Telephone/standing	1.4	1.6	1.8	2.0	2.2	2.4
Typing						
electric	1.4	1.6	1.8	2.1	2.3	2.6
manual	1.6	1.8	2.1	2.4	2.7	2.9
Waiting in line	1.3	1.5	1.7	1.9	2.2	2.4
Wallpapering	2.4	2.8	3.3	3.7	4.1	4.6
Washing clothes, machine	2.1	2.4	2.7	3.0	3.3	3.6
Washing dishes, hand	1.8	2.0	2.2	2.4	2.6	2.8
Watching TV	1.1	1.3	1.5	1.6	1.7	1.8
Woodworking	2.6	3.0	3.4	3.8	4.2	4.6